The International Library

PSYCHOANALYSIS AND SUGGESTION THERAPY

Founded by C. K. Ogden

The International Library of Psychology

PSYCHOANALYSIS
In 28 Volumes

PSYCHOANALYSIS AND SUGGESTION THERAPY

Their Technique, Applications, Results, Limits, Dangers and Excesses

WILHELM STEKEL

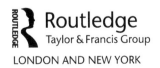

Routledge
Taylor & Francis Group

LONDON AND NEW YORK

First published in 1923 by
Routledge, Trench, Trubner & Co., Ltd.
2 Park Square, Milton Park, Abingdon, Oxfordshire OX14 4RN
711 Third Avenue, New York, NY 10017

First issued in paperback 2014

Routledge is an imprint of the Taylor and Francis Group, an informa business

© 1923 Wilhelm Stekel, Translated by James S van Teslaar

British Library Cataloguing in Publication Data
A CIP catalogue record for this book
is available from the British Library

Psychoanalysis and Suggestion Therapy
ISBN 0415-21107-7
Psychoanalysis: 28 Volumes
ISBN 0415-21132-8
The International Library of Psychology: 204 Volumes
ISBN 0415-19132-7

ISBN 13: 978-1-138-87570-8 (pbk)
ISBN 13: 978-0-415-21107-9 (hbk)

Wenn jemand alle glücklichen Einfälle seines Lebens dicht zusammen sammelte, so würde ein gutes Werk daraus werden. Jedermann ist eigentlich des Jahres einmal ein Genie. Die eigentlich sogennanten Genies haben nur die guten Einfälle dichter. Man sieht also, wie viel darauf ankommt, alles aufzuschreiben.—LICHTENBERG.

[If one could assemble in compact form all the happy ideas that have occurred to him in a life-time the result would be a good work. Everyone is really a genius at least once a year. The so-called geniuses simply have the good ideas occurring to them more closely together. Thus it is evidently highly desirable to write them all down as and when they occur.]

TRANSLATOR'S PREFACE

In this work Dr. Wm. Stekel not only outlines in telling strokes the working technique and the practical applications of the New Psychology, a field in which the author ranks as one of the foremost masters and pioneers, but the uses of various other forms of psychotherapy, including the much-discussed method of hypnosis, are also given and defined.

The author's emphasis is laid on the end-results of the various methods of treatment. The busy practitioner and the nervous sufferer who seeks advice because he earnestly means to get well are alike interested in the first place in results.

Another characteristic feature which distinguishes this work from all other introductory treatises is the instructive, clear-cut manner in which the author, on the basis of his own experience with the various psychotherapeutic methods in vogue, points out the limitations of each and the dangers of excess. It is most helpful and highly instructive to find one of the pioneers discussing so frankly the limitations and the possible dangers of psychoanalysis. That is a much-needed lesson, and it should save many an over-enthusiastic beginner from regrettable errors or excesses.

Translator's Preface

In addition to the true scientist's candor, Dr. Stekel displays the qualities and skill of a born teacher in the manner in which he treats the various practical problems relating to the practice of psychotherapy. The volume is not only a reliable guide : in the midst of the many over-enthusiastic works on psychoanalysis and psychotherapy for beginners, it stands out as a timely corrective, and I am, therefore, glad to provide an English version of this much-needed warning by a master-hand.

JAMES S. VAN TESLAAR.

Brookline, Mass.

CONTENTS

Contents

PART I

TECHNIQUE AND APPLICATIONS
OF PSYCHOANALYSIS AND
PSYCHOTHERAPY

PART I

TECHNIQUE AND APPLICATIONS OF PSYCHOANALYSIS AND PSYCHOTHERAPY

In its early stages the technique of psycho-analysis was very simple. Breuer in 1880 achieved a remarkable therapeutic success with a patient, partly through a sort of autohypnosis and partly through ordinary hypnosis, after overcoming her hysterical amnesia. Several years later Freud again took up this work. Starting with the assumption that those affected with hysteria suffer from painful reminiscences which they are unable to get rid of or " abreact " (the reminiscences in question being experienced during a sort of " hypnoidal state " only) Freud, after hypnotizing the patient, attempted to rouse his memories of the repressed traumatic incidents, thus drawing these experiences into the field of consciousness, and accomplishing a complete "abreaction." The earliest results favoured this treatment, as shown in the *Studies of Hysteria* by Breuer and Freud, which appeared in 1895.

But this method of treatment soon proved insufficient for the investigation of the " un-conscious " processes. The fact that many neurotics—among them, those suffering most acutely from compulsions and anxieties—could not be hypnotized, the uncertain nature of hypnosis, and that it is not always possible to maintain the proper *rapport* with the hypnotized subject, induced Freud to improve his technique. He discovered—and this is perhaps his outstanding, most ingenious achievement—the " technique of free associations."   The patient was not questioned. He was merely asked to relate everything that came into his mind, and to be very careful not to overlook the smallest detail that might occur to him, even though it should seem to him to have nothing whatever to do with his case.   In his first technique Freud used a method which he has long since abandoned, but which is still employed by Bezzola and by Frank (by the latter in connection with hypnosis).   If nothing occurred to the patient's mind, Freud would press his hands against the patient's forehead and assure him that something would presently occur to him.   This device was very helpful in lessening resistance and filling out disagreeable pauses.   However, Freud soon became convinced that this method also served to cover up the resistance, and he therefore gave up the plan of forcing the reminiscences to the surface.   A pause in the patient's account of his experiences indicated an inner resistance which must be recognized and overcome before the analysis of the neurosis could proceed successfully.

The technique eventually adopted took the following form : The patient stretches himself comfortably on a sofa ; the physician seats himself at the back of the patient and allows him to give unrestrained utterance to all his thoughts just as they occur to him, the physician having first familiarized himself with the nature of the complaint, through an accurate account of it.

This technique has been modified by many practitioners of psychoanalysis. For my part, I cause most of my patients to sit facing me, since many find lying down unpleasant. But I admit that the method suggested by Freud has certain advantages, and is the only possible method with a certain class of patients. During a free conversation, the patient finds it easier to conceal his resistance to the disclosing of the " inner complexes." That resistance is more plainly recognized when the patient lies down and Freud's technique is rigorously followed.

Jung has adopted the association experiment. He notes the patient's answers to certain " stimulus words " and from the delayed reaction to some of these words he derives a knowledge of the emotionally stressed "complexes," a term signifying the "constellation of a number of images." That method has no practical value, but is of great utility in scientific and psychological research. More practical is my method of causing the patient to utter a number of words (without stimuli) as they occur to him. Usually these words (one or several) bear some relation to the complex which the patient is hiding from me.

For years, however, I have not used this technique at all, as I am of Freud's opinion that the uncovering of the inner resistance is the first task of psychotherapy : both Jung's association method, and mine, conceal these resistances instead of revealing them.

I refer so frequently to resistance that I must first explain their nature. Briefly expressed then : Every patient clings to his neurosis. This neurosis is to him a convenience in life, a protection against the evil world, and has come to represent a part-fulfilment of his phantastic wishes. He cannot do without his neurosis. He is afraid of good health and suffers from the "will to illness." Perhaps non-analysts, who are sceptical about a "will to illness," will understand me better when I say : The neurotic lacks the will to get well. This is a truth which we find most difficult to grasp. Only through psychoanalytic experience do we come to fully appreciate the almost incredible fact that the patient is enamoured of his illness. He is proud of his ailment, and makes use of it as a means of insuring his power over his environment or of avoiding some unpleasant duty (work, care of the sick, unwelcome visits, etc.). I here give an account of the psychoanalysis of a veterinary surgeon who came to me to be treated for a very distressing " acathisia " (inability to sit down). For three years he had been troubled with this complaint. The trouble most seriously interfered with his practice, which was chiefly in a rural district in the neighbourhood of a small town. He was unable to remain seated in a carriage, had to drive standing, and so on. The analysis brought prompt relief. He was soon cured, was able to sit down, and all the distressing neurotic symptoms disappeared. When he was about to return home cured, he confessed to me that he " was really sorry to be cured." He had that day heard an inner voice whispering to him : "Keep up your illness ; it is so interesting to be an invalid."

In order to appreciate the resistance of patients to their recovery, we must understand the nature of a neurosis. Every neurosis is the result of a mental conflict. Thoughts so unpleasant and painful, as to be unbearable to consciousness, are driven out of it, or rather, driven in, in the technical psychoanalytic expression, repressed. If the mental conflict were clear to the patient, he would not become neurotic ; he would merely be unhappy about it. We can appreciate the statement of Freud that " We can only convert hysterical unhappiness into real unhappiness." But this is rather too pessimistic an outlook. By disclosing the root of his trouble to the patient we may point out to him the road to the kingdom of health and happiness. This task requires psycho-pedagogic re-education. The analysis must not and cannot be an end in itself. " Psycho-pedagogy must go hand in hand with psycho-analysis."

With these rather meagre facts in hand, let us now proceed to a psychoanalysis in order to learn the technique of the science, by the use of a practical example.

We will return to the veterinary-surgeon already mentioned, who suffered from acathisia.

At the first interview he told me the history of his trouble. He belonged to a good family, showed no hereditary taint, was the son of well-to-do parents. His health had always been

good except for the usual illnesses of childhood.
A careful physical examination (which must
never be neglected) showed nothing abnormal
with the exception of "vagotonia." His trouble,
(acathisia) had been going on for three years.
It developed slowly : at first there was but a
feeling of discomfort when sitting down, so that
he often fidgeted or changed his place. Gradually there developed paresthesia, attended with
pain. The pain was slight at first, but soon
became so intense as to be unbearable. He was
unable to sit down. If he attempted to do so,
he felt such intense pain that he cried out. He
tried all sorts of things to ameliorate his
condition. He had all the seats of his chairs
upholstered. That relieved him for a few days,
and then the trouble was as bad again as ever.
He next tried the plan of having the seats of the
chairs cut out so that nothing should come into
contact with the sensitive parts.* This, like
everything else that was suggested and tried,
proved ineffectual. The physicians differed in
their diagnosis. X-rays were taken, but they
proved negative. An operation had been
suggested by a surgeon (resection of a nerve),
but to this he would not submit, because a
satisfactory result could not be guaranteed.

* The pain came then from the pressed parts.

He was, I think, on the point of committing suicide, unless I could help him. Morphine and all other drugs, hydrotherapy, electricity—all proved equally useless in the end. He doubted whether psychoanalysis would achieve anything. He believed himself to be beyond help —that his case was hopeless. Had I ever heard of such a strange case ? Surely he must be the only being with such " an unheard-of " trouble.

The next day the psychoanalysis began. I advised him to tell me everything that came into his head. I cautioned him against omitting anything that occurred to him, no matter how trivial it seemed—he was to tell everything. The patient was silent for a few moments ; then said : " Ask me questions. I would much rather ! " That is typical. The patient does not like the method of free association. He does not know what to say. This attitude has its reasons. Neurotics are dreamers, and to a certain extent addicted to double thinking. They live in a world of phantasy, and have lost the habit of keeping, as it were, in close touch with their own train of thought. They are distracted, and never attentive to what is going on within them. They are unable to concentrate. Psychoanalysis means training in concentration—it is a schooling for the observation of one's own thoughts. The patients must be led to it. Therefore they are told: " You must tell all your thoughts, even when they are unpleasant, even when the thoughts are about the physician himself, doubting or depreciating him."

Certain medical circles still hold to the erroneous view that psychoanalysis is a painful ordeal, a sort of spiritual inquisition, a continuous interrogatory. Precisely the reverse is true. A question might divert us from the complex and lead us entirely astray. Naturally questions are occasionally asked. But the questions always bear some relation to the matter introduced by the patient. In the psychoanalytic conduct of a case it is impossible, for instance, to predetermine that we shall deal, on a particular day with sexuality, and on the following day with the subject of pride, and on the next with " the feeling of inferiority." The patient is the one who leads, even though he must be kept under control, as we shall fully explain in our next chapter.

Having given this necessary explanation, we now return to our patient. He gave his reminiscences, but with reluctance and hesitation, and mentioned several physicians who had promised him a cure, only to disappoint him.

By this I perceived that the patient desired to express his first doubts regarding the efficacy of psychoanalysis. The resistance had begun and was directed against the physician and his method. Finally he said how much his wife suffered on account of his condition, that she had become very nervous, and that he was more worried about her than about himself.

At this juncture I asked a question about their marital relations, and was told that for several years past the patient had had no intercourse with his wife, that he was absolutely impotent, that he was too sick a man to think of such things. He had morning erections, but when he approached his wife the erection promptly subsided. He was absolutely impotent with her.

I at once suspected that his trouble was in some way connected with his marital relations, but I avoided suggesting anything of the kind in my questions.

The next day the patient appeared five minutes late. Usually that in itself indicates a resistance, although the subject may assert that the street car was to blame. But I reflect that he has a whole day in which to get ready for our appointment; I know that other patients, whose resistance is not so great, arrive an hour before the appointed time rather than be one minute late. I am familiar with the various excuses intended to cover the resistance. I may, therefore, look for but little progress in the analysis that day, and in this I am not mistaken. The patient began to talk about psychoanalysis and tried to drag me into a learned theoretical discussion on the subject. He wanted to know precisely how the unconscious can influence the pain, and so forth. Such theoretical discussions should be avoided, as they lead nowhere. We must abstain from trying to convince the patient with arguments, merely pointing out that the psychoanalyst's case will be proved by the success of his treatment. The patient then advanced as his next opinion that my contention that dreams have meaning and are of use in psychoanalysis cannot be correct. That on the previous night he had had a trivial dream which certainly could have had no sense in it. I ask him to tell me the dream. At first he was unable to recall it. The dream had been nothing but a mass of nonsense. Mere repetitions of some of the day's happenings. Finally—upon my insisting—he did recall the dream-picture. He said: " My wife was speaking to the servant-girl, and made a very disagreeable face. She was reproaching the girl with leaving the rooms in disorder. She also pointed to a little bottle. I said : ' Leave the girl alone.' What else happened I can't remember."

Since the dream awakened the patient, it must have been attended with great emotion. As to the meaning of dreams and the technique for their interpretation, I must refer the reader to my book entitled *The Language of Dreams* (translated by J. S. Van Teslaar, and published by the Gorham Press, Boston). At first the patient was unwilling to attribute any meaning or significance to this dream. It was merely the repetition of incidents that had occurred on the previous day, trivialities such as took place almost daily in his household.

His wife disliked that servant, but he found her indispensable in his business. She knew all his routine and his drugs, helped him to clean his instruments, and was extremely reliable. He had had to intervene repeatedly between his wife and the girl. Although he loved his wife dearly and could not imagine life worth living without her, he abhorred this bickering, and was beginning to be harsh to his wife in spite of himself.

Incidentally he repeated that he had had no sexual intercourse with his wife for months past, because he was impotent with her, that he felt no desire, that she was like a good comrade to him, but otherwise left him cold.

From that point onwards the analysis proceeded more smoothly. Slowly the picture of the family relations unrolled itself before my vision. I heard that he had passed through a period of bitter jealousy over his wife. She had once cried out in her sleep : " My God ! Why do you make your sausages so different ! " and then she repeatedly cried out : " Heinrich, Heinrich, I want to die now ! " He wakened her, and pressed her to tell him the truth. He had for a long time suspected that she had, during their engagement, been unfaithful to him in her intimacy with a student. Now that suspicion had crystallized into a certainty. The wife, thus pressed, was driven remorsefully to confess her guilt. After that their home became a hell. He tortured her with his jealousy, wanted to know all the details of the intimacy, and threatened her with divorce, a step which he kept deferring out of consideration for the children. During that very period his wife roused his passion tremendously. Every quarrel ended in renewed intercourse with her, during which he was tortured with the thought that she would have enjoyed it more with the other man. His passion knew no bounds ; he felt as if he wanted to chain her to himself ; and he then discovered for the first time how much he loved her.

But slowly a change had set in. The satyriasis turned into impotence. He became more quiet, though still entertaining thoughts of revenge. The seducer was employed as a forester at a half-day's journey from his home. He thought out plans how he might lie in wait for the forester and shoot him dead. He wanted to do it in some way that would divert all suspicion from himself. He was very fond of hunting, and was in the habit of using his spare time in roaming through the woods. He thought how easy it would be to shoot his enemy from behind. He would waylay him towards sunset and shoot him down from an ambush. Once he had been on the point of carrying out his plan, but his hand had trembled so violently that he was unable to discharge the weapon.

At this point the analysis might be discontinued. In the neurotic we have discovered the criminal ; we have laid bare a psychic conflict between the consuming passion for revenge and the fear of the law—and of God's punishment. The patient is a religious man, who attends Church regularly, and who has absorbed into his very flesh and blood the idea of sin. But he is also a creature of impulse. His strong religious feelings serve as a protection against his instincts. He must be pious in order not to falter.

But we are thinking of the dream and of the puzzling incident with the servant-girl. His wife had shown the girl a small bottle. What does that bring to his mind ?

He hesitated, and then resumed his reminiscences. He had been fond of the girl for a long time : but he had indulged in no familiarity with her until after his wife's confession. Finally, the girl had become his mistress. Now he was impotent with his wife, whereas in the girl's company his potency asserted itself at once. In his intercourse with her he had the strongest orgasms he had ever experienced. He loved the girl and could not live without her. He was also jealous of her, and for his sake the girl had had to give up a lover, who now pursued him and had threatened him with revenge. He had also received anonymous letters. His wife had also received anonymous letters calling her attention to the affair. Since then there had been no peace in the home. The wife requested him to discharge the girl. The girl demanded that he should send away his wife, divorce her, and marry herself instead. But he could live

2

neither without the girl nor without his wife; he saw no way out of the dilemma.

These statements of fact did not clear up the meaning of the little bottle in the dream. But this detail was cleared up a few days later. The patient declared that the thought had once suddenly occurred to him that he might poison his wife. She had once drunk the contents of a little bottle of Cherry-bay with suicidal intent. It occurred to him, whilst giving her injections, as he often did in the treatment of her attacks of gallstone colic, that he might use a large dose of morphine or some other deadly drug, and thus end the conflict. But the thought had only flashed across his mind for the fraction of a second, and had always been dismissed from consciousness. On the contrary; moral reaction led to the reawakening of his affection for his wife, to the arousing of a certain sense of pity for her, and now he was more than ever convinced that the advent of death or any separation from her, who had always been a kind and cherished helpmate, would be a calamity he could not survive.

This, then, was the serious conflict from which there seemed to be no escape. He stood between two women, equally in love with both and unable to live without them. But his thoughts secretly revolve around one point : " If your wife should die now ! Then you would be free and could enjoy the girl without molestation, while you must now be content with such embraces as you can enjoy with her at hasty and stealthy rendezvous." The ideas of getting rid of his wife were not eradicated. They had only been forced back into his subconsciousness. Now his fear of sitting becomes clear. It is a symbolic fear. It means : " I have the fear of being locked up for my crimes " —he plays with two murder obsessions—" of being compelled to sit."

We might now consider the analysis finished. With this insight and knowledge of the patient's inner relations, the discomfort of sitting should have disappeared. The pain had, in fact, diminished considerably, but it had not disappeared altogether, although he was able to sit down for short periods. The patient had meanwhile realised that he could free himself from his conflict only by adopting a radical treatment —the only possible one under the circumstances : he must discharge the girl and live with his wife. What had partly helped to drive him from his wife's into the girl's arms was his craving for revenge. He knew, too, that the girl's fiancé would gladly marry her. Our patient had to learn to look at his wife's mistake with humane eyes, to forgive her, and on the basis of that forgiveness, to begin a new life with her. This is where the educative influence of psychoanalysis begins.

But the pain did not disappear. Further determining elements of the symptom had to be sought. We must gradually learn to appreciate the fact that the neurosis builds up its systems in the course of an attempt at a compromise, so that various factors, forbidden and tolerated tendencies, guilt, lust, and punishment become fused into a single symptom.

The neurotic symptoms settle preferably in the *locus minoris resistantiæ*. But they also readily seize hold of some *erogenous zone*. Frequently the *locus minoris resistantiæ* is an erogenous zone. The sensitive organ may be the seat of sexual feelings.

The patient had had trouble with his posterior parts for some time past. As a student he had a slight periproctitis ; later he had suffered from hæmorrhoids, for which he had had to be operated upon and which also had been diagnosed as the cause of his later trouble. His fæces were hard ; he had to sit long and strain hard at his stools.

It is not possible to go into every detail here of the course of the psychoanalysis, of how resistances were overcome which had perceptibly increased under the influence of the new revelations. It became manifest that the patient had strong homosexual tendencies. During his youth quite a number of transitory homosexual episodes had occurred, which had afterwards been entirely forgotten. Homosexual acts were now disgusting to him. But we psychoanalysts know that disgust is but the negatively toned craving. Any one familiar with the law of " bipolarity of all psychic phenomena " which I have formulated (called by Bleuler " ambivalence ") will not be surprised at these mutual correspondences. He will look upon disgust as the product of the repression of a craving which is unbearable in consciousness.— So much, in brief, for an understanding of the case.

Further analysis revealed a strong homosexual leaning towards the servant-girl's fiancé. I discovered only after four weeks of analysis, that the young man in question had been in the patient's service as coachman, that he had been called to the colours, and that thereupon my patient, taking advantage of the situation, had taken his place with the servant-girl. He asserted that he had already told me these facts. This is a favourite subterfuge among neurotics when they are off their guard and blurt out some unpleasant revelation. They at first fancy they have told us these things, and in the end believe that they have actually done so.

I next discovered that my patient had often seen the coachman naked, and had admired his private parts. I then heard for the first time that "much to his astonishment" he had dreamed of indulging in homosexual acts with that coachman. Any one who, like Näcke, in his book *Der Traum als feinstes Reagens auf Homosexualität* (The Dream as the most subtle reagent of Homosexuality) recommends the use of dreams for diagnosis, might be inclined to look upon this occurrence as a proof that our patient was homosexual, but he would discover that he had made a serious mistake. Like all neurotics and, in fact, like everyone else, my patient was bisexual. Only the neurotic's bisexuality is more pronounced, and when disappointed in love he reverts to his infantile sources of pleasure—a process called by Freud "regression." My patient was afraid of any contact with buttocks and neighbouring parts, because such contact, by association, rouses the underlying homosexual wishes. The pain or discomfort serves the purpose of emphasising a pleasurable feeling, as I have repeatedly pointed out. I have quoted a number of examples in my *Nervous Anxiety* (London, Kegan Paul; New York, Dodd and Mead, 1923). But I was surprised to learn that this neurotic symptom yielded a certain amount of secret gratification, although it was not a conscious pleasure, but assumed the guise of pain. However, the neurotic symptom enabled the patient to concentrate his thoughts on the erogenous zone, the anal region ; it made daily exposure of the parts before physicians and bath-attendants necessary ; and thus gave him opportunities for gratifying his fairly marked " exhibitionistic " tendencies.

In its larger outlines the case may now be considered finished. Various other infantile thoughts came to the surface, but their discussion here would lead us too far afield.

The effect was prompt. The acathisia disappeared altogether—the patient went home cured. The girl was at once dismissed ; in fact before his return home, and she married the coachman, who went to live elsewhere.

The cure may be credited to the psychoanalysis or some may attribute it to the power of suggestion. One thing is certain : psychoanalysis has given us a deeper insight into the mental mechanisms of this neurosis than would have been possible with any other method.

Psychoanalysis and suggestion are opposites. What do we understand by suggestion ?

At a time when everybody is talking of suggestion, when the stage is filled with hypnotizers and the tendency is to explain everything by suggestion, and when suggestion is made the subject of public discussion, the phenomenon remains misunderstood, and every unusual psychic process is ascribed to it. There are mystical, metaphysical, physiological, telepathic, spiritualistic, and magnetic explanations given, as Isserlin points out in *Bewegungen und Fortischritte der Psychotherapie*, in *Ergebnisse der Neurologie und Psychiatrie*, vol. I, Jena : Gustav Fischer, 1912.

Bernheim says ; " Suggestion is that process through which an idea is introduced into, and accepted by, the mind." That, of course, is no explanation, no definition—merely a description. According to this view, the teacher's explanation in the class-room, perceived and " taken in " by the pupil, is also suggestion. Bernheim, indeed, seems to admit as much, for he goes on to say : " Every impression, every mental picture, every fact of awareness is a suggestion." From that standpoint the whole process of learning consists of suggestion, and it would be difficult to explain why some particular suggestion should take deep root whilst another did not.

Dubois says : " Suggestion is an inspiration or prompting which takes places in secret ways."

By this Dubois means that suggestion escapes the critical faculty. This antithesis to the psychic constellation is emphasized also by Trömner, whilst Vogt lays particular stress upon the " unwilled and uncontrolled development of the roused tendency." But these definitions, too, attempt to explain the nature of suggestion without accounting for the suspension of the critical faculty.

L. W. Stern's definition is : " Suggestion is an art of transferrence whereby one person assumes another's mental attitude as his own." This explanation comes somewhat nearer to the nature of the process. It points out that another's mental concept is perceived by the subject as if it were his own. But how—and why ?

Lipps gets still nearer the truth when he emphasises the effect of the imagination : " Suggestion is a process whereby, under proper conditions, influence is exerted by rousing the imagination." He goes on to say : " Every suggestion requires the presence of the hypnotizer, and his success depends on his ability to win the trust of the subject, on his power to insinuate himself into his confidence, and thus to dissipate every doubt and every thought of opposition or contrariness." This definition presupposes that the suggestor's will-power will be stronger than that of his subject. Suggestion which, according to Janet, is an automatism of the split psyche, a function of the partial self according to Lipps, means submissiveness to a stronger self-conscious personality.

Bleuler was the first partially to solve this problem when he taught us that " Suggestion is an affective process." It is not the thought, nor the imagery that triumphs—no, it is the feeling or affect which is transferred and carries the thought along with it.

If the teacher is capable of rousing his pupils' interest, he is listened to attentively, and is able to exercize suggestive influences over him.

But what is the character of the interest which the suggestor must rouse in order to be able to transfer his thoughts ? Let us revert to our school example. If the pupil likes the teacher, the latter's teaching finds ready access to his soul. He must honour and respect the teacher, admire him, worship or love him—in other words, he must believe in him. The teacher must be able to rouse his pupils' emotions.   Suggestion, therefore, is the transferrence of an emotion—a process whereby the suggestor "fascinates" the subject.

But what is here understood by fascination ? It is a sudden feeling of love and sympathy.   To love means "to find one's God."   At the moment of suggestion the suggestor becomes the God who has to be blindly obeyed because the subject believes in him implicitly.

We live in an expectant mood, momentarily awaiting some marvel.   We have never really given up our belief in miracles.   The old beliefs of our childhood in the supernatural, in those endowed with magic power, still secretly linger in our soul.   In our infancy our parents had seemed to us to be wonderful, to be endowed with all that was great and good, omniscient, all-powerful, possessed of magic gifts.   Time dispels these childhood thoughts.   Our parents are the first to lose their divine attributes in our eyes, and with them the glory of the entire world fades away.   In his autobiography, Hebbel tells us of his absolute faith in his father's omnipotence, until one day, during a terrible storm, he saw him fall trembling on his knees and anxiously lift his hands in prayer to God.   Not until then did the boy realize that there was a being higher even than his father. Until then his father had been his God. But the first emotions in the child-soul survive in us forever. " Alles erste ist ewig im Kinde," says Jean Paul Richter (" Every first thing is eternal in the child "). The faith in our parents is indestructible and remains with us to the end.

Two forces dominate our souls : The will to power and the will to submission. So powerful is the latter that it is manifest even in the most independent souls among us. Love is the will to submission. Our submissiveness in the reception of a suggestion is no testimony to the strength of the suggestor, but rather to our own weakness. We submit, not because he wills it, but because *we* do, just as we fall into a natural sleep because we wish to sleep.*

For example : The suggestor says energetically : " You cannot raise your arm ! " We try to do so and do not succeed. The will to submission has taken away our will-power, which, now in the service of the suggestor, commands us to believe his words. We become as children who lose their own will-power in relation to their father. Suggestion is therefore a sudden regression to the infantile state, and the

---

* Cf. My monograph: *The Will to Sleep* in *Twelve Essays on Sex and Psychoanalysis* (New York, 1922).

emotions of faith, love and awe are mobilized within us. Every human being carries within him many fractional souls, among which is the child-soul. The child within us desires to witness a wonder : it cherishes the illusion, and submits to the power of suggestion because that becomes part of its actual wish. We do not want to lift our arm. It would be untrue to say : " We cannot lift our arm." *Nicht : wir können nicht wollen, sondern wir wollen nicht können* (" It is not that we will not because we cannot, but we cannot because we will not ").

The healthy person is more amenable to hypnosis than the neurotic, who has raised all sorts of barricades around the self of his childhood, and finds submission more difficult on account of inhibitions and fears, as well as on account of his habitual attitude of stubbornness and rebellion. The healthy person submits because he does not think such a reversion to infantilism possible.

But what has the analysis to do with suggestion ? Had I assured the patient that all would be well when he had freed himself of his complexes, we should be justified in suspecting the influence of suggestion. But I had promised no cure. I had only suggested a trial.

Suggestion does not take into consideration

the causes or deeper motives of the trouble—on the contrary, it is an arbitrary, a forceful interference with mental processes, whereas the analysis investigates the psychic roots of the neurosis, lays them bare, and shows the patient what is really troubling him ; it compels him to recognise frankly those conflicts which he had up till then pushed aside from the sphere of his consciousness ; it trains him to attempt a final solution of his trouble.

We will now return to our patient. The acathisia enabled him to vacillate between his wife and the servant-girl, and to indulge, during his quasi-unconscious states, in his criminal phantasies. I enabled him to take a dispassionate view of his thoughts, to give up the repression, to overcome his criminal tendencies, and to make up his mind definitely to settle his conflict by discharging the girl and thus freeing his soul. I brought about the change from his sheltering himself under the guise of illness to his return to health.

The question may be raised : Might not the same result have been obtained through suggestion ? Hypnotize the patient, interrogate him about his complexes, tell him what he cannot or does not wish to know, and in a few days the case might be cured, whereas, with your method, it takes two or three months to accomplish the same purpose.

To this I answer : " Quite apart from the fact that it is very difficult to hypnotize neurotics of this kind, they do not disclose their complexes under hypnosis. I have hypnotized thousands of hospital cases of traumatic neuroses. With the exception of pronounced simulators, most persons, and particularly the healthy (a fact I wish particularly to emphasize) are easily hypnotized. Secondly, cases of traumatic hysteria are easily subjected to hypnosis. But anxiety-neurotics, compulsive neurotics, impotents and hypochondriacs, are almost insusceptible to hypnosis, and when in that state they are hardly approachable. There are, it is true, some few exceptions to this rule. Moreover, this particular patient had tried hypnosis and Dubois' method, but without success.

The hypnosis covers up the resistance ; it accomplishes no educational task ; it gives us no insight into the psychic structure of the neurosis. In opposition to Frank, Warda and Loewenfeld, I must emphasize this point. Hypnosis and psychoanalysis are opposites.

I must here add a few remarks on the nature and technique of hypnosis and fascination, and on the treatment of war-time neuroses.

Every neurologist has his own method of treating the neuroses, and has achieved the desired end if he has put his will into it. A cursory review of the works which have been written about the war-neuroses shows that most physicians have relied upon the faradic brush (electricity) as the panacea for troubles of this nature. The technique has varied, but has amounted, in most cases, to the same thing—leading the patient to forego his complaint on account of the discomfort caused by the therapeutic application of the electrical brush. The neurosis is in its essential character the fixation of an affect. In the post-war neuroses that affect was the anxiety induced by fear of the battle-front, or the inner repugnance to the duty of serving. We have seen severe neuroses manifesting themselves in uncontrollable shivering fits, on account of which those suffering from them could be employed only in auxiliary services (such as watchmen or in the A.S.C.), especially when the sufferers found that the trouble entitled them to the benefits of hospital treatment. Every proper kind of treatment is bound to arouse a counter-affect. Fear of the pain caused by the faradic brush pushed the fear of the trenches into the background. But a feeling of pride may give rise to similar miracles.

Suggestion is the transference of an affect (Bleuler). The affect thus transferred breaks up the neurosis affects which serve as the nucleus for the growth of the symptoms. The transferred affect may sometimes be faith in the physician, or love of him. That forms the basis of the good results obtained by various neurologists who employ narcosis following an appropriate suggestive preparation of the patient. It thus depends to a certain extent upon the psychic disposition of the physician himself whether he accomplishes his results through fear or by inspiring love and confidence.

I have chosen the latter method, and have found it to yield excellent results. I have been able to effect a cure, in the end, with every case that had not been subjected too long to other methods. I have seldom used psychoanalysis, usually limiting myself to hypnosis and fascination, and very often to suggestion during the waking state, a method whose technique is very simple.

Speaking generally, it may be said that nearly every hospital patient is susceptible to hypnosis. But this is true only of patients in the military hospitals, where their attitude of submissiveness towards those in authority favours the method. In private practice the conditions are not nearly so favourable.

I must point out another fact, as yet recognized by very few nerve-specialists, and that is, that healthy people are the most favourable subjects for hypnosis. There are certain neuroses which render the subject unapproachable. I count among the latter the more severe forms of the compulsive neuroses and the anxiety-neuroses. Experience has also taught me that a person can be more easily hypnotized in the presence of a number of people, e.g., in a hospital ward, than when alone with the physician. That is because patients are always uneasy lest something unpleasant may happen to them. An hysterical female patient, might fear a sexual assault, and therefore be unable to fall asleep if alone with the physician. In fact, she is capable of imagining a sexual assault during the hypnosis, when this is not true, because she enters the physician's consulting-room imbued with the phantasy that such an assault will take place. It is therefore advisable to refuse to resort to hypnosis except in the presence of others.

The favourable results reported by Nonne in post-war neuroses I am, on the whole, able to corroborate, and I may also add that I have always found it possible to hypnotize, even foreign-speaking patients, with the aid of an interpreter. It suffices to have taught them beforehand the sentence " Now you must go to sleep at once," or briefly the command " Sleep." Of course, hypnosis is easier if the patient's language is known. But, in opposition to the statement of Wagner-Jauregg, my experience has been that those of the Slavic race—even when the physician is unfamiliar with their languages —are far more susceptible to deep hypnosis than others.

In my hospital practice a single case, among some six hundred, proved refractory. That was the case of an advanced simulator, a case that was easily solved later on. But hysteria is not simulation. It is playing at illness with one's self, a flight into illness—the final result of " unconscious " forces.

My technique used to be the simplest imaginable. I looked at the patient steadily for a few seconds, and then commanded him in an authoritative tone : " Sleep ! " Usually the nurses or other patients had prepared him for what was coming. An atmosphere surrounded him favourable to the treatment. I caused deaf and dumb patients to witness several hypnoses ; I then looked them steadily in the eye and uttered a couple of sounds. They invariably repeated the sounds in a state of " fascination," and the trouble was soon cured.

Hypnosis in some cases leads to satisfactory results. I employ that method when I want to avoid psychoanalysis, a treatment which I reserve for the more serious cases. The psychotherapeutist should not be one-sided: he should adapt his method of treatment to every case with a view to its special conditions —in other words, he must individualize his method of treatment. There are cases in which the dialectic method of Dubois—persuasion— is best; others to which hypnosis is most suitable. Psychoanalysis I reserve for the cases which prove refractory under the other methods and which require a longer period for re-education.

The question, now, suggests itself: Which cases are suited to psychoanalysis? How far does the realm extend within which psycho-analysis may be found useful?

Originally Freud applied his method to a very restricted field; he regarded only hysteria and compulsion-neuroses as psychogenous disorders and as curable by psychic means. He draws a distinction between "actual neurosis" (*Aktual-neurose*), brought about through some disorder of the sexual life, and the "psychoneuroses" proper—the so-called "transference-neuroses" which are traceable to repressions. The actual neuroses are : neurasthenia, anxiety-neurosis, and certain forms of hypochondria. Anxiety-neurosis is brought about through *coitus interruptus*, or some other deleterious form of sexual indulgence. So-called neurasthenia, according to Freud, forms a sharply defined clinical picture. Its symptom-complex includes : dull headache with a feeling of pressure, spinal irritation, dyspepsia with flatulence and constipation, paræsthesias, diminished potence and depression. This form of neurasthenia, in Freud's sense, is the result of excessive masturbation. He states: " Neurasthenia is always traceable to a condition of the nervous system such as is brought about through excessive masturbation or which results spontaneously as the result of frequent pollutions ; anxiety-neurosis always betrays sexual influences characterized by premature withdrawal or unsatisfactory gratification such as *coitus interruptus*, abstinence in spite of strong libido, or so-called frustrated excitation. (*Sammlung kleiner Schriften zur Neurosenlehre*, vol. I.)

According to Freud's earlier contention, the phobias, too, belong to the category of " actual neuroses." He denied their psychogenesis. In his essay on Anxiety Neurosis (*Sammlung*, vol. I) we find the following statement : " In the phobias of anxiety-neurosis the affect is monotonous—(1) is always anxiety ; (2) it does not owe its origin to a suppressed image but on the contrary proves itself, upon psychological analysis, irreducible further, so that it is not amenable to psychotherapy. The mechanism òf substitution, therefore, does not hold true for the phobias of anxiety neurosis."

These views I strongly opposed, even whilst I was a member of Freud's immediate circle. I denied the existence of " actual neurosis " without psychic causation, and shattered the hypothesis that all anxiety-neuroses are psychically determined and not amenable to psychotherapy.

The first case of " agoraphobia " (fear of public places) which I had occasion to treat was that of a cashier in one of the larger banks. I was able to prove that he was entertaining the thought of escaping to America with a sum of money—in other words that he was under the domination of an unconscious " idée fixe " in the sense of Janet, who, with his keen insight, had reached a fairly correct understanding of these unconscious processes.

After uncovering this criminal impulse at one sitting of the patient, he gave up his position as cashier at the bank, and the trouble disappeared without further analysis.

The second case was that of a woman who was unable to appear in the streets unless accompanied by her husband. I found that the husband was absolutely impotent ; that the woman was constantly struggling against thoughts of temptation ; that she required the presence of her husband as a protection against her pressing unconscious temptations (cf. my monograph *Causes of Nervousness*, authorized English version by J. S. Van Teslaar). I have formulated the following generalization: " Every neurosis is the result of a psychic conflict." I have been able to trace the underlying conflict in numerous cases of so-called neurasthenia and anxiety-neurosis, thus furnishing the missing link in the chain of evidence that *all* neuroses are, contrary to Freud's contention, psychogenetic.

Freud, at first, doubted the diagnosis. My cases of anxiety-neurosis were, in reality, cases of hysteria. But I was able to show him that he himself had made the diagnosis " anxiety-neurosis " before the cases had come under my care. He then proposed that these psychogenetically determined cases should be called " anxiety-hysteria," and the cases without psychic causation " anxiety-neurosis." I accepted that *sacrifizio dell'intelletto*, against my better judgment.

Freud now seems willing to recognize the psychic origin of actual neuroses, as I gather from Hitschmann's very instructive survey of Freud's teachings (Hitschmann, *Freud's Theory of the Neuroses*, translated by Dr. C. R. Paine ; London, Kegan Paul and Co., Ltd. ; New York, Moffat, Yard and Co. 1921).

The analysis must aim at reaching its goal in the shortest time possible. It achieves its aim most quickly in the actual neuroses. The latter are the neuroses in which the conflicts date from a relatively recent period. A girl forsaken by her betrothed after a three years' engagement, loveless, lonely, disappointed, and becoming depressed as a consequence, needs only the psychotherapy involved in appropriate consolatory talks. In such a case profound analysis, even though the condition be a serious one, would be superfluous, and under certain conditions may even prove harmful. And that is, *mutatis mutandis*, true of all the neuroses induced by a conflict of recent origin. The case is different when we deal with neuroses in which the conflict depends on an exaggerated sense of pride, a disproportion between ambition and ability (*wollen* and *können*). In the latter case, psychoanalysis must include psychopedagogy— a system of re-education through psychic means

—the two must go together. It is part of the physician's duty to help the patient to overcome his morbid feelings, and to correct his false attitude towards life.

Prognosis is favourable in anxiety-neurosis ; the condition is curable in from four to six weeks. The compulsive neuroses prove refractory in about one-third of the cases, and require a somewhat longer period. In these disorders psychoanalysis is the only appropriate method, because it is the only method which takes cognizance of the psychogenesis of the condition.

Excellent results are achieved in cases of psychic impotence, when verbal suggestion is often all that is necessary. More frequently a certain amount of analysis is required, but never the aid of hypnosis. On the other hand, sexual anæsthesia in women is more difficult to overcome, though it, too, is a most promising field for psychoanalytic endeavour.

The various forms of hysteria require longer treatment—sometimes as long as half a year. Stuttering is curable in a short time. The results are excellent.

Startling results are also achieved in the treatment of epilepsy (see next chapter) a condition which I was the first to treat by psychotherapy, and to prove amenable to that form of treatment. But I know no more difficult task, and would only entrust it to very skilful and experienced psychoanalysts.

Thus far I have indicated but a small portion of the field in which psychoanalysis and psycho-therapy generally may be successfully applied. Among the disorders easily curable by these means may be mentioned cases of headaches (so-called neurasthenic and hysterical headaches) head-pressure, inability to work, inability to concentrate, neuralgia, baffling " rheumatic " pains, asthma of nervous origin, constipation, tics, writer's cramp, vaginismus, nervous stomachic disorders, cardiac neuroses, etc.*—in short, all the disorders which indicate a psychogenous (neurotic) component (treated fully in my work, *Anxiety States*).

A tremendous field for psychoanalytic endeavour is furnished by the various neuroses of sexual life—the sexual perversions, which Freud has described as being retained infantilisms, but which he unfortunately has not investigated further psychogenetically. According to Freud " The neurosis is the negative of the perversion." My professional experience has taught me to investigate the perversions—which I call " para-

---

* *Vide* Stekel, *The Nervous Heart;* ibid. *The Nervous Stomach;* both translated by J. S. Van Teslaar.

phillias "—also, as neuroses. This I have extensively proved with regard to homosexuality (*vide Bi-Sexual Love, The Psychopathology of the Homosexual Neurosis*, Pt. I, authorised version, by J. S. Van Teslaar. Boston, U.S. : Badger). Homosexuality is curable through psycho-analysis, but only when the patient earnestly desires to be cured, and is willing to give up his sexual feeling-attitude—a condition which, unfortunately, is rarely met with. But the record of a number of successfully treated cases justifies a psychoanalytic attempt whenever conditions appear favourable.

I was the first to disclose and describe the psychogenetic origin of the complicated con-dition known as fetishism (*vide Zur Psychologie und Therapie des Fetischismus—Zentralblatt f. Psychoanalyse*, vol. IV, 1914, also *Störungen des Trieb-und Affektlebens*, vol. VI : Fetischismus, Vienna : Urban & Schwarzenberg, 1923). The prognosis is favourable. The duration of treat-ment is at least four months in the more compli-cated cases, in which the revulsion against woman has been carried to the extreme point, so that sexual gratification is attained only through substitution of the fetish.

Morphinism, cocainism, dypsomania and similar troubles also fall within the province of psychoanalytic therapy, for they are always psychogenetic ; *hyperemesis gravidarum* (excessive vomiting during pregnancy), fainting fits, dizziness, shivering fits, paræsthesias, muscle-cramp, and the anxiety-neuroses of children have also proved favourable fields for psychotherapy.

I wish to call particular attention to the satisfactory results obtainable with stubborn, unmanageable children, whenever these traits are not due to psychopathic inferiority, but are the result of neurosis. Wonders are accomplished in such cases, especially if the children are removed from their usual environment, against which their neurosis is chiefly directed. The parents themselves are often neuropathic subjects, and in a certain sense, largely responsible for the children's neuroses.

The treatment of the psychoses raises a much more formidable question. I have observed some rather encouraging results in melancholia. During the earlier stages good results are often attained but cyclothemia is apt to be unapproachable. During the analysis of a maniac depressive we are likely to find the depression-phase setting in, possibly induced by the taking up of the unpleasant complexes.

Paranoia, during its earliest phase, may occasionally, though not always, be corrected. Bjerre has reported such a case ; I myself have had two favourable cases, in one of which the treatment is not yet completed. But, on the whole, I am not inclined to advise any psychotherapist to expect great results in the treatment of the psychoses. Often we find so-called " affect-psychoses " being mistakenly treated for " dementia precox." The prognosis is favourable in the " affect-psychoses " ; eventually these conditions may yield to treatment enough for the patients to return to their work, whereas genuine dementia precox—called "schizophrenia" by Bleuler—has so far proved almost wholly incurable, even though the psychic structure of the condition be readily discernible. The attempt may be made, but the family should be warned of the hopeless outlook ; and should be made to understand beforehand that it is but an experiment and that a cure is well-nigh hopeless.

These are, in broad outline, the limits of psychoanalysis as a therapeutic procedure. I suggest, however, that every psychotherapeutist should take up a case at first for one week's observation, and not until he has done this determine whether the case is suitable for psychoanalysis or should be given up. There are patients suffering from neuroses that are decidedly psychogenetic but who nevertheless defy every form of therapy. They have settled down into a policy of a " dual life " : they do not want to know anything at all about their unconscious or subconscious trends ; they may have some conception of what these processes are in others, but are blind regarding them in their own case, and resent the least attempt to approach their own inner mental life. Such cases must be left to their fate.

There are other cases in which the suspected neurosis proves actually to be a psychosis, though this may not be discovered until after from ten to fourteen days' observation. In these cases I call the attention of the other members of the family to the fact that the patient's trouble is a psychosis, and decline to go on with the treatment, refusing to take it up again, except at the express wish of the family and with the clear understanding that neither cure nor even amelioration may be definitely looked for.

Unless this precaution is taken, psychoanalysis may afterwards be blamed for the outbreak of the psychosis, the inimical attitude of professional psychiatrists contributing in no small degree to this end.

It is highly desirable that physicians shall acquire the necessary knowledge of psychotherapy, and particularly that they should become familiar with psychoanalysis. Departments for instruction in psychotherapy and in sexual science are necessary, and the two divisions should by preference be placed under the control of one and the same specialist.

The present educational situation with regard to these subjects is unsatisfactory. It is unfortunate that physicians still pass through special schools without being trained in these most important branches of their profession. The time will come when sexual science and psychotherapy will be represented in the curriculum of all medical schools and students will be trained and examined in these most important branches. The fate and welfare of numberless patients depend on the adoption of these measures.

Psychotherapy has its legitimate field precisely as pharmacotherapy. It may have an even greater future.

I trust that this little contribution may help to draw the attention of the profession to these pressing needs.

PART II

THE FINAL RESULTS OF
PSYCHOANALYTIC TREATMENT

50 Psychoanalysis and Suggestion Therapy

Dies stete bespiegeln und Auskundschaften unseres Selbst—wohin führt es ? Der Gedanke tritt zwischen den Menschen und das Leben, und verbrennt die Früchte die es bietet. [This continuous mirroring of ourselves and our self-scrutiny—whither does it lead ? Reflection breaks in between man and his life, and destroys the fruits that the latter offers.]
—HEBBEL.

PART II

THE FINAL RESULTS OF
PSYCHOANALYTIC TREATMENT

I

EVERY psychoanalyst finds that it is very difficult for the patient to reconcile himself to the discovery of his hidden instinctive cravings. If the analyst is careless, and discloses too much of the cryptic interplay of forces during the first consultation, he awakens thereby the patient's resistance against the treatment, and as a result the patient is likely later to absent himself under one pretext or another. Sometimes the greatest care is of no avail in this respect. The fact is that the patient first enters the physician's consulting-room with the determination " not to give himself away." Every neurotic guards the secret of his neurosis as a precious possession, as his special treasure, of which he must not allow himself to be deprived. If he scents danger for his pet fancies he takes refuge in flight. . . . The greatest precaution is often powerless to prevent this. In a couple of days or so the patient will suddenly discover that he is already cured and take his leave, with profuse declarations of gratitude to the physician, not forgetting to add that he will recommend the treatment to some of his relatives and friends. . . . As a matter of fact, he is no better than he was at the beginning. Another will be suddenly called away on an unexpected journey; a third discover that the treatment is " too exciting " for him, and that he must quiet himself down before he goes on with it ; and so on. There are endless variations to the excuses conjured up. It is well, therefore, to enter upon each case with a considerable amount of scepticism and with the greatest care. The more the doctor keeps his trump cards and his knowledge to himself, the more certain is a favourable result to ensue. It is foolish to offer explanations to the patient during the first stages of the treatment, even should he appear to be well-informed on the subject of psychoanalysis and perhaps a physician himself. The reverse is the fact. Those well-informed are the most difficult patients to treat. They are forewarned, and use their knowledge of psychoanalysis to organize resistances against the psychoanalysis. I therefore absolutely agree with Freud, who advises against the plan of lecturing to the patients with a view to explaining psychoanalysis to them or in the expectation of thus aiding the progress of the treatment.* At first sight it might seem as though this might hasten the cure. The patients read psychoanalytic writings eagerly, and thereby learn ways of concealing their inner self against the physician's attempts to disclose their unconscious tendencies. It is foolish to allow patients to read everything. I did this whilst I still believed that the patient had a genuine desire to be cured. Now I know that the neurotic is animated by but one dread, i.e., the fear that he will get rid of his neurosis. One of my compulsion-neurotics in the course of the analysis developed a new dread, this very fear of " losing something." It turned out that the root of that feeling of dread, was the fear of getting rid of the neuroses and of becoming well.

The psychoanalyst who prepares his patient with preliminary talks is like the strategist who delivers into the enemy's hands his plan of at!ack. Therefore I only allow my patients to read general, superficial accounts of the subject. One of my patients studied psychoanalytic

* Freud, *Ratschläge für den Arzt bei d. psychoanalytischen Behandlung* (*Zentralbl. f. Psychoanalyse*, vol. II).

literature day and night, with the alleged intention of hastening his recovery. When I objected to this plan, he met my remonstrance with the statement that when doing so he recalled various significant incidents. These reminiscences he then carefully noted down so that the consultation hour was hardly long enough to cover the ground. But all this was farcical, and, in spite of his endless notes and reminiscences, he only hovered over the surface of things.

We cannot proceed successfully towards the prosecution of our aim until we have learnt to appreciate this effort on the patient's part in its true light. The greatest measure of resistance does not depend on the transference, i.e., on the patient's " falling in love " with the physician, as we once thought. The transference is but a form of resistance. Every psychoanalysis betrays a tendency to switch the attention of the patient away from the past and from the neurosis proper by concentrating it on the present moment. Every patient is inclined to interrupt the consultation with numerous accounts of his present complaints. Sometimes patients will even say : " As long as I don't get this off my mind there is no use in trying to continue ! " The consultant should

not permit these tactics to obscure the issue.
Whenever the danger is impending that the
nucleus of the trouble may be disclosed, these
minor complications break in. One of the
most potent factors is the transference, the
attachment to the physician. What is the use
of talking about the emotional fixation on the
father when there is, so to speak, a present
emotional attachment to be dealt with ? This
attachment to the physician may be used as a
means of promoting the patient's recovery. For
neurotics never get well for their own sake.
They get well to please the physician. They do
it as a favour to him.

II

It is now some years since I first pointed out*
that a patient's first dreams often display his
resistance symbolically, and with irresistible
strength.

A patient submitted to me the following
dream :

" I am standing at the teacher's desk in front
of the blackboard, on which I see the following

---

* *Darstellung der Neurose im Traume* (*Zentralbl. f Psychoanalyse,*
vol. III, No. 1.;

drawing. My task is to solve the problem mathematically, or by means of drawing, and I feel quite helpless. Lamp-light."

The patient draws the picture as follows :

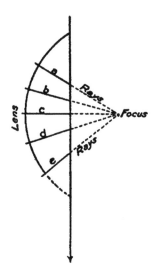

The analysis of this dream reveals a number of determinative factors. It would be very tempting to explain the patient's whole neurosis on the basis of this dream. But I must limit myself here to my present theme. The patient showed me the drawing with the light marked by points. " Here the picture ends," said the patient, pointing to where the rays break off. He merely has the feeling that behind the wall there is a source of light. The dream indicates that the source of the neurosis must remain undisclosed. The five rays, on first association, remind him of five girls with whom he had been in love at different times ; Ray *a* is thickest ; then the rays grow successively dimmer, so that ray *e* is rather vague. All the five girls become fused into one picture. They revert back to one central point. I found out afterwards that the central point in question was his mother. In other words, the five girls were surrogates for the only genuine love of his life . . . the most recent was the strongest love affair. But ray *e* was nearly forgotten.

But what is the meaning of this first dream as a whole ? Plainly, that he does not propose ever to disclose to me the whole truth. The analysis will only lead up to a certain point and there stop. The physician who, in this dream, is represented as the examining teacher, will never find out the whole truth. The patient will only penetrate as far as the superficial layers of his mind ; his memories and thoughts will reach no farther.

I pass by the other determinations of the dream as irrelevant in connection with our immediate subject. I only want to point out the unfavourable omen which the dream casts upon the treatment. And the patient actually behaved as the dream foreshadowed. His memory only carried him to a certain level, beyond which he found himself unable to go. But, as the dream-analysis revealed, against his will the whole extent of his complexes, particularly his unconscious homosexuality (burning point=anus), he suddenly discovered all sorts of excuses for taking refuge in flight. Before that, he had diligently studied, though against my advice, everything on which he could lay his hands that bore on psychoanalysis, in order, as he asserted, that we might get along more rapidly with the analysis. As a matter of fact, this was but a means for learning how to cover up his neurosis with various defences. He studied diligently the plans and strategy of his antagonist—the psychoanalyst. Three months later he returned, determined to take up the struggle anew. For he was chiefly interested in winning a victory over the psychoanalyst and in bidding farewell to the physician without having been understood or cured. In a few days he brought me the following dream, which plainly disclosed his new attitude towards the struggle :

" I am standing with my brother in front of my new house, and am keeping sharp watch. A couple of thieves appear ; I point my revolver and shoot. I hit one in the back. I think to myself : ' Oh, this is unpleasant—how shall I prove that I acted in self-defence ? ' "

I pass over the obvious homosexual meaning, and turn my attention to the resistance displayed in this dream. The new house is his new neurosis. He had built a new house during my absence. The brother also figures as a symbol of his neurosis. I myself am one of the thieves (the other, according to the patient's associations, is Freud), and I am trying to break into the dark chamber of his soul. Here we have the functional symbolism (Silberer) in its wonderful plasticity. He cannot act in any other way. He must defend his neurosis and protect himself with all the means at his disposal, against my skill in the art of breaking through. . . .

In another dream this patient saw a certain professor Jodl swimming with powerful strokes in a basin of water. He was ordered to follow the swimmer, and did so, reluctantly, and presently stopped the professor. The basin represented his soul. Jodl, a professor of psychology, stood for me. The end of the dream was that he swam back alone. The dream revealed his jealousy of the analyst, his attempt to surpass the latter, and to accomplish his own cure unaided.

III

The deeper I penetrate into the nature of psychoanalysis, the stronger is my conviction that the analysis really means a continuous struggle with the reluctant patient, who is, at heart, unwilling to get well, even though he pathetically avers the contrary. The illness is generated expressly for the purpose of enabling the patient to dominate his environment and to carry out his will, though at great cost to himself. The patient is therefore antagonistically disposed towards the analyst from the very beginning. His own fate comes to be a secondary consideration. For the time being, the physician stands as a symbol for the whole world. The patient aims at winning a victory over his father and over his teacher and over his whole environment by defeating his analyst. If he does get well, he does it to please the physician. But instances of this kind are relatively rare. In most cases the patient is disposed to deride the physician's efforts, and intends to come out victorious in the end. Even sufferers from *impotentia*, who complain so bitterly of their misfortune and avow that they would be the happiest people on earth if they could only get rid of this handicap, meet the physician's efforts with considerable inner resistance.

The " will to power " is the neurotic's all-powerful trend. And that " will to power " means, " Above all, I want to be loved." . . . Will to power is will to be loved. The patient endeavours in every possible way to induce his physician to love him. He even goes so far as to lead the way by proffering love, and does not disdain to beg for love in return. He at first yields to the sway of his will to subjection and falls in love with the physician, who, in the course of this emotional transference, is made to play all sorts of rôles.

His own final object is always borne in mind by the patient from the beginning of the treatment. To begin with he does not wish to prove an easy case. When I first began practising psychoanalysis I was naïve enough to think that I was doing the patient a favour when I told him that his case was not a serious one, and that I had treated others like him. Every neurotic looks upon his neurosis as an extraordinary work of art, an ingenious structure securely protected by numberless walls and moats against the incursion of any enemy ; hence he is incensed at the thought of having to share his invention—the product of his genius—with others. An easy cure would, of course, prove that his ailment was of a trivial character—and that he is by no means willing to admit, or to allow others to believe. I once treated a physician who had retired from practice and had had to return home. I had been treating him for four months. He chanced to meet a man who had been under treatment by Freud for over a year. This made him angry, and he wasted a month's time brooding over his disappointment at the thought that his own case had been cured so much more quickly. Why had the other man required a whole year ? Was not his a more serious case ? Perhaps I had under-estimated the seriousness of his condition, and so forth.

This example illustrated in a very instructive manner the analysis of the transference. Some psychoanalysts believe that dissolution of the transference means drawing the patient's attention to the fact that he is emotionally attached to his physician. In most cases, nothing is gained thereby, and the patient remains as closely attached as before. Dissolution of the attachment means the uncovering of the parallel constellation which has detached from its moorings an affect not yet abreacted or cleared up, but still operative. Furthermore, it means revealing the resistance which that situation generates instead of allowing it to remain concealed under the emotional transference. That is what happened in the case just mentioned. The patient's father did not believe that his case was very serious. And as I stood as substitute for the father, my belief that his case was not a serious one, and that a few months of treatment would effect a cure, roused great anger and resistance on his part. During the stage of transference I stood in the place of the father.

I will turn now to another case to illustrate the meaning of transference. I recently treated a patient to whom I proposed that we should carry on our talks whilst walking out of doors—a form of treatment which I have found highly efficacious in some cases. But this particular patient was unable to recall any associations, and remained peculiarly silent during our walks. He preferred to stay indoors, where he " felt much better." It turned out that in his youth his father had often compelled him to join him on walks and the recollection of these unpleasant compulsory excursions with his father acted as a resistance during the transference. The old attitude of contrariness against the father was revived by the parallel situation.

We see, therefore, that psychoanalysis may reawaken the old relationship of opposition between father and son, between the older generation and the new. The struggle with the physician arouses the old feelings of antagonism endowing them with new strength and life. Presently it will lead the patient to adopt the attitude of supremacy over his physician, and to part from him victorious in the end. We must not forget, either, the pleasure conferred by the neurosis itself. What can we offer the patient in its stead ? Realities which, in contrast with his fancies, must appear to him to be pathetically inadequate substitutes.*

I may add a few remarks concerning the nature of transference. To love a person means to understand that person. To be loved means to be understood. If the patient is confident that the physician understands him, he will love him. We must not forget that most neuroses are disorders of the love-affect. He who heals their troubles must be capable of giving the patients the supreme medicament for which they are yearning—i.e., love. The transference of that love from the sexual to the erotic realm,

---

* I must refer the reader to the exhaustive account of a case of impotence (No. 103, p. 339) in which this struggle continued for six years, until finally, with my aid, the patient triumphed over his former physician.

and its transposition into the ethical standards, often requires the highest skill on the part of the physician, who may easily succumb to counter-affection.

IV

In my larger work, *The Dreams of Artists* (authorised English version by J. S. Van Teslaar) I have exposed and described the neurotic's faith in his " great historic mission." The skill with which neurotics cover up this faith, and how they struggle against giving up the fiction, are difficult of belief. What is the value of reality when compared with the alluring phantasy of their great historic mission ? The neurotic is an apostle ; he is God's anointed ; he has hitched his waggon to a star ! The whole world will some day admire him and prostrate itself before him ! The world may scorn and scoff at him now, but he will yet triumph over all ! And the struggle with the physician becomes a replica of his struggle with the world at large. He measures his forces against the physician's, and fights for the right to retain his neurosis. For, we must repeat, he does not really want to get well. He seeks all sorts of reasons for this *Wille zur Krankheit*. For instance, a neurotic may fear that the analysis may interfere with his creative ability as a writer, yet he may never have accomplished anything as an author. His very neurosis may have attained such depths as to render any creative activity impossible. One neurotic told me in all earnestness that he feared the analysis might foster a tendency to perversions in him. . . . . Another brought me the following dream at our first session : "I am lying on a sofa. Kornitzer arrives, and is very tender towards me. I say to him : 'Now you have come to me, but it is too late. I do not want you now.' "

Kornitzer had been a former colleague with whom he had been on friendly terms until they parted on account of business-differences. It is easy to see that there was a certain homosexual tension between them, and that Kornitzer here stood for myself. In the dream he lies down on the sofa, as he does during the progress of the psychoanalysis. [His was one of the cases in which the reclining posture favoured the flow of the association of ideas.] And yet this dream contains a deeper meaning : it betrays a rationalized resistance. I ask him whether Kornitzer is good looking : "The very picture of health," the patient answers promptly. Kornitzer, then, is also the picture of health in the dream—translated, the dream means : What

is the use of the treatment ?   Health has been
too late in coming.   If I were younger there
would be some sense in it.   But—at my age !
Yet the man was only thirty-five years old.

This undercurrent of resistance suggests to
patients all sorts of objections to psychoanalysis.
One patient declares himself tremendously
interested in the art of dream-interpretation.
He brings so many dreams with him that it
would take years to analyse them.   The dreams
give some indications of the trend which the
physician has suspected from the very beginning.   But there is trouble ahead for the
inexperienced analyst, who may be led thereby
to declare : " We shall soon discover the
important trauma in the situation ; we are
getting nearer to it."   The dream-chase then
begins in earnest.   Each dream appears to be
more interesting than the previous one.   The
trauma is dramatized in the most varied forms
and pictures.   The associated thoughts come
nearer and nearer to the significant traumatic
incident.   Months pass by—but the sought-for
nucleus does not reveal itself—it was not there
at all !   The patient was playing hide-and-seek
with his physician.   Within himself, the neurotic
will smile and feel triumphant over his physician's
helplessness and shortsightedness.

V

The misuse (due to misunderstanding) of the notion of sexual trauma is extraordinarily widespread. For years I have held that in and of themselves the traumas mean nothing, and that incidents are raised to the quality of traumas by the neurotic. The traumas seem to retain an actual determinative power only in the case of certain forms of " psycho-sexual infantilism " (fetishism, exhibitionism, etc.). Usually such traumas are fully conscious. Members of the Vienna Psychoanalytic Society will remember that I once facetiously declared that for certain children traumas are the best form of sexual enlightenment. The trauma acts thus only within certain definite constellations and on the basis of a physical predisposition—a fact which Abraham had already pointed out. Elsewhere I have described the significance of sexual traumas in the life of the adult. It would almost seem that children easily shake off the effects of traumas. For while these traumas of children are exceedingly frequent, they are relatively rare among the real determinative factors in the etiology of the neuroses.

Indeed, we see children who experience numerous traumas, and who nevertheless remain perfectly well. The neurotic has the tendency to scrutinize the past critically, and to search for incidents on which to fix his consciousness of guilt. He also needs to find occurrences independent of his will and hence serving as excuses. The " Tendency to find excuses for himself " plays a great rôle in the dynamics of the neuroses. The trauma frees the patient from the troublesome self-reproach with which he has surrounded his neurosis. He transfers his responsibility to some traumatic episode. Some traumas act as perpetual moral admonitions. It is a striking fact that most neurotics are able to relate their traumas at the first consultation. We used to think that this was exceptional : but it is the rule. The neurotics know their traumas, and many attribute to them their troubled state, from the very first. This is especially true of those patients who are familiar with Freud's doctrine of the neuroses. Indeed, sometimes neurotics begin with the sceptical remark : " I don't see how psychoanalysis is going to help me. I know my traumas ; I know my repressed thoughts—in fact I have none at present. I am quite aware of my incestuous tendencies. . . . Consequently, what can I expect psychoanalysis to do for me ? " Physicians especially those who themselves practice psychoanalysis, are likely to assume this attitude and to evince that obstinacy, with reference to their own complexes, which I have called "psychoanalytic scotoma." Among them are to be found some rather keen-witted, well-trained minds. But in matters pertaining to himself the cleverest of men may be rendered stupid by an affect.

In his *Vorlesungen zur Einführung in der Psychoanalyse* (Vienna : Heller, 1917) Freud gives us a synthetic account of his latest views regarding his doctrine of the libido. According to this account, the libido strives to become attached to some object in the external world. If its course is interfered with—in other words, if the individual finds he is unable to find external gratification of his erotic cravings—the libido becomes dammed up. It reverts to various infantile positions, and through this reversion the old infantile traumas again acquire significance. This is said to be the origin of the psychoneuroses which Freud, following a suggestion made by Jung, calls "transference neuroses" (*Übertragungsneurosen* " i.e., hysteria and compulsion-neurosis) ; or else the libido reverts to the person's own self, this giving rise to the narcistic neuroses (dementia præcox, paranoia—the latter called by Freud paraphrenia

—and melancholia). As the libido endows the
infantile unconscious traumas, it flows back
into the unconscious. The task of the analysis
is, therefore, to dissolve the fixation upon childhood, to release the unconscious, and to
facilitate a new fixation of the libido upon its
proper external objects, or its sublimation into
spiritual values.

Here we again have the doctrine of the
significance of the infantile traumas, which has
caused so much confusion in psychoanalysis.
Freud has recently emphasized the significance
of trauma. In his latest contribution, *Aus der
Geschichte einer Infantilen Neurose (Sammlung
kleiner Schriften zur Neurosenlehre*, 4te Folge.
Vienna : Heller, 1918) he again attempts to
prove that an infantile sexual trauma was the
cause of a serious neurosis. The trauma in
question was not disclosed until after three years'
exploration !

Without attempting to belittle the significance
of infantile traumas, I can only state that the
case as published did not seem to me convincing.
In previous writings I have expressed myself at
length regarding the disadvantages of such
protracted periods of treatment. I strongly
suspect that many neurotics are tortured for
years with questions about their sexual traumas.

The histories of those cases which I have published, and the prompt results obtained, at least show us that it is possible to attain to a satisfactory insight into the depths of a neurosis, and that, therapeutically too, the best that we ought to expect, may be achieved without overstressing the infantile factors. I could not have accomplished more than this, had I prolonged the treatment over a course of three years. The duration of the treatment in individual cases was from a few days, a few weeks, to, at most, three months.

VI

There are, of course, a number of cases in which certain repressions are first disclosed through the analysis. But in most cases the patients relate things which they have always known and have not wanted to disclose. Thus, for instance, one neurotic did not describe her compulsive ceremonial (mannerisms) to me until after six months. She had, in fact, mentioned it before, but she had done it so superficially and imperfectly that she had not given a true conception of the situation.

Another compulsive neurotic did not describe his mannerisms (ceremonial) on defecation to me until after a year's treatment. This is the patient to whom I owe the clearest and deepest insight into the pliancy of the neurosis. I must frankly confess that I did not learn to appreciate the dynamic power of resistance until I came into contact with this case. He did not want to confess his defecation-mannerisms to me. He wanted to triumph over me. He wanted to prove himself the stronger. He did not want to get well. I was at the time still under the spell of Freud's doctrines, and I believed that a compulsive neurotic could be cured only after a prolonged course of treatment (one year or longer). Now I achieve that result in three or four months, even in the most severe cases of compulsion-neurosis.

I know of patients to whom inexperienced psychoanalysts have promised a cure as soon as their infantile traumas should be disclosed. Thereupon there has followed a wild chase through their dreams. Dreams were brought up daily which referred to some trauma. The physician was triumphant, " Now we are near the trauma ; we shall soon have it now." But the patient's secret victory was greater than his doctor's. He was merely leading his physician by the nose. He produced the most artful dream-constructions, which the physician finally had to reject as artifices. This went on for four months. The patient stayed at home all day long wracking his brain to recall his reminiscences. He reproached himself very seriously for not co-operating better. The physician on his part dissolved transference after transference, yet the analysis did not progress any farther.

. . .

What we must specifically bear in mind is, that patients are really not keen to get well. With their tongues they clamour for a cure, but their actions prove the reverse.

It is not easy to induce a patient to give up his neurosis. The dissolution alone is not enough. Sometimes the patient permits the dissolving of a symptom, thus lending a semblance of reality to his alleged desire to get well, and permitting the physician a slight triumph. The emotional transferences may be accomplished without following the devious and troublesome path of psychoanalysis. That is why certain slight forms of neurosis may be readily cured by a superficial psychoanalysis. But this, too, may be sometimes accomplished by other means. The fact is that it is not the method, but the physician who heals. Psycho-analysis enables us to penetrate more deeply into the structure of the neurosis proper. It lays bare before us the patient's resistance to his complete recovery. It discloses his antagonistic attitude, his perennial readiness to assume the offensive—an attitude which is at the same time a defence.

Considerable ingenuity and experience are required to penetrate through these disguises, to release the patient, and to free him from his contrary inclination.

Bearing in mind these various considerations, we are led to recognize the fact that the ending of a psychoanalytic course of treatment is one of the most difficult problems. The best prognosis is yielded by those cases in which the attendant circumstances permit only of a relatively short time for the treatment. The employee with but a couple of months' vacation at his disposal, the physician who has to interrupt his practice, people who make great material sacrifices for the sake of their health, these are the people particularly anxious that the treatment should take as short a time as possible. The problem is much more difficult in the case of wealthy, independent people who seem never to want to get through with it. Their struggle with the physician becomes more important to them than the ultimate result of the analysis. They will forgo the prospective cure, about which they are but luke-warm, if they may only triumph over their physician ; they would rather be able to maintain the attitude : " You may have cured a great many others, but you cannot deal with my case so easily. In fact, you cannot cure me at all."

I treated a wealthy man for a serious neurosis, whose one refractory symptom was a fear of public places (agoraphobia). In every other respect he was cured. His gastric disturbances, his attacks of indigestion, his social reticence, his inability to work, had all been overcome. But, in spite of all my efforts, his agoraphobia did not disappear. He interrupted the analysis unexpectedly, and returned to his former physician. The latter advised him to go to an oculist who was curing troubles of that nature by prescribing glasses. In fact, the doctor accompanied the patient on the journey to Germany to consult this particular oculist. And what did this faithful patient say, when in the train ? Why ! characteristically enough he declared : " It will be the greatest triumph of my life to know that Dr. Stekel did not absolutely cure me—that he could not—that I shall owe my complete recovery to some one else ! "

The glasses helped him for a few days, but soon the old trouble returned. He was disinclined to attribute the victory even to his family physician. The next thing was that he heard about a masseur, who undertook to cure him in a few days by massage. As a matter of fact, he was able to walk about the city freely after only three applications of massage. He was completely cured. He owed his recovery to a simple masseur, and thus scored against all his professional advisers.

VII

If we take these peculiarities in our subjects, into consideration, certain matters become quite clear to us. We can understand the results obtained in certain sanatoria with patients who have previously undergone a psychoanalytic course of treatment. Many an opponent of psychoanalysis takes pride in the fact that he has in a short time cured cases which the psychoanalyst was unable to cure after a prolonged course of treatment. But these gentlemen merely reap where others have sown.

We can easily understand why our erstwhile patients become our most inveterate antagonists, fighting us with scientific arguments and with slander. The final result of the analysis discloses the true character of the person analysed.

A person of real delicacy of feeling will not lend himself to such procedure in spite of the inner urge, but those of a different temperament, such as we often meet in the course of our psychoanalytic practice, will just as certainly follow out their lower impulses.

On the other hand, we may console ourselves with the obvious fact that our good results are *de facto* far-reaching and much more effective than they appear on the surface to be. For many patients who leave us apparently uncured, do, after a short period of incubation, effect a self-cure, or are healed by some other physician, sometimes even by some quack.

Nearly all patients dread the termination of the analysis. I will here point out only a few of their devices to show how diplomatically the psychoanalyst has to conduct his cases in order to parry his patients' subterfuges, with even subtler tact.

A woman, who had been under my care for about half a year on account of a fear of public places (agoraphobia) was apparently well and ready to return home. She could go some distance without fear or anxiety, and she fully appreciated this improvement in her condition, for she had been troubled for thirty years with this difficulty, and during that time she had been

unable to travel, or to go out at all, even with
an escort. A few days before her departure she
experienced a tremendous attack of dread while
in the streets. She came to me very discouraged,
and told me of her plight. How could she go
home now, before she was really well ? I made
it clear to her that this was a case of uncon-
sciously seeking a reason for prolonging the
treatment and for remaining in Vienna. Her
anxiety-attack had developed in order that
she might need a continuation of the treatment.
Her next dream was as follows :

" I had given my old shoes to my aunt and
was standing naked and barefoot. I thought
to myself : ' How can you now go into town ! '
and I dreaded having to go through the streets
without my shoes on. . . ."

The aunt in question had been dead long
since. She had been a poor woman, and had
received small gifts from the dreamer—possibly
a pair of shoes. The patient related that she
was fond of walking barefoot, and lately she had
often been surprised to find herself starting out
without her shoes. Here we find clear indications of foot-fetishism, such as are frequently
met with among neurotics suffering from disorders of locomotion. But the explanation of
the dream as an exposition of my patient's

neurosis yielded the following result : The old shoes were very large and yet they pressed her feet. Indeed, they had irritated her feet across the insteps. The shoes were the symbol of her neurosis. She was about to transfer the neurosis—to make a present of it—to her deceased aunt, that is, to bury it with the dead, and to attempt to live without her neurosis. But she had lived with her neurosis for thirty years. The illness caused her discomfort (shoe pressure), but it was to her a sure defence against the uncertainties and dangers of life. . . . Now the task she had to face was to go through life without the protection of the neurosis. She dreaded it. Another determinant led associatively to my name. Shoe-heels are called here, colloquially, *Stöckel*. She needs low *Stökel*. This is a pun on my name. In short, she is unable to get along now without my protection, my advice, my suggestions. The dream portrays also a desire for freedom, like many of the later dreams of those who are cured. I am thrown aside with the dead.

Now began the hide-and-seek game on the patient's part. She wanted to be well, and yet was afraid to be well. If her emotional attitude be motivated largely by contrariness she will cling to her agoraphobia. The situation was further

complicated by the patient's inability to free
herself from me. At such a stage the doctor
must have the will and determination to break
off the analysis as soon as the chief motives of
the patient's anxiety have been revealed and the
patient sees clearly the relationship between the
feeling of dread and these cryptic motives. The
patient, under the circumstances, may return
home dissatisfied, but after having tried some
other cure, will often, without taking any further
steps, shortly begin to walk about freely. This
was the condition of the patient that I have
described in Chapter XXI of the second, and
Chapter XX of the first edition of my *Conditions
of Nervous Anxiety*.* The treatment was interrupted after four weeks, and the patient left in
an improved condition. I met her walking
along on the *Ring*, without escort—a thing she.
had previously been unable to do. She admitted
that shortly after giving up the treatment she
began to improve without having recourse to
any further remedies. The patients feel that
they are protected by their neurosis. One of
my patients called his neurosis his *Gehschule*.
. . . The physician becomes to them the
substitute for their neurosis. Eventually they

* Authorised translation by R. Gabler. London : Kegan Paul
& Co ; New York : Dodd, Mead & Co., 1923.

have to learn to do without their neurosis and without its substitute, the physician. That is a tremendously difficult task for those who have lost all power of self-reliance. . . .

To return to my patient who could not walk. She had measured her strength against mine all along. She now had to face the necessity of giving up the treatment and of acknowledging herself conquered. That was beyond her power.

VIII

Anyone who becomes familiar with the hidden structure of the neuroses cannot but recognize the justice of Adler's contention when he speaks of a fictitious goal which the patients seek as the aim of their underlying motives. I have found that this fictitious goal is Heaven and eternal bliss. In the case of the woman under consideration, her whole neurosis was directed towards safeguarding herself against temptation and insuring for herself eternal happiness. She intuitively felt she was too weak to follow the straight and narrow path of virtue, and therefore she thought of insuring for herself eternal bliss in the next world through her dread of open spaces in this. What

were to her the joys of this world compared to
heavenly bliss ? Her one object was to reach
Heaven. I believe her whole life was a preparation for the supreme test before her God. She
hoped that all her privations would be so many
points in her favour and must increase her
chances of eternal bliss. She also manifested
a belief in her " great historic mission "—a very
wide-spread fiction among neurotics. She was
no ordinary person—she was holy, God must
take special note of her, and must mark her for
special treatment. In short, she made herself
as snug within her neurosis as the proverbial
" bug in a rug," and thus protected herself
against the crude realities of everyday life. She
no longer cared to walk about. Among other
dreams she had the following : " I am going
out, and rejoice at the thought. Then I cannot
find my pretty knitted jacket, so I have to stay
at home. I might otherwise catch cold."

The knitted jacket is the web of her neurosis.
She cannot live without her neurosis. She is
afraid lest the beautiful ardour of her faith
should cool, and so she wanted to prolong the
treatment.

I assumed a bellicose tone. I told her that
" I had decided to discontinue her treatment,
that she might return to her home." The

indignant woman pointed out that other women who had suffered from a similar agoraphobia had been under my treatment for a longer time.

" True," I answered, " but the outlook was more encouraging. Those patients used to come to me, unaccompanied, after the first few weeks. If you would come to me by yourself, I should be more hopeful as to your prospects of a cure, and might then consider the question of continuing your treatment. Your fear of open spaces is not the neurosis, but only a visible symptom of it. . . ."

Three days later the woman came to me unaccompanied, and since then she has been walking about the streets freely without any fear.

I pressed for an early termination of the treatment. The woman hesitated, and, as it turned out later, with good reason. There were still some things she had to tell me. There was another feature in her emotional attitude which had to be corrected. She was anxious to triumph over me and disclose my incapacity. She brought me the following dream : " I scolded my servant because she had only half-cleaned the kitchen. In one half of it there was a lot of dirt lying about ; the other half was clean."

That kitchen was a symbol of her soul, or, if you prefer, a symbol of her brain, and the

neurosis was being swept out of it. I had not
done the work thoroughly. I was the servant girl
in the dream. I was her hired servant. She
gave her orders, and I was to obey. In short, her
pride would not permit me to end the treatment.
She wanted to be the one to do that when
she thought the proper time had come. It
was her privilege to give notice to her hired help.
She then brought forward a mass of additional
material information, which she declared she
had already told me. This was again an
artifice to belittle me and to triumph over me !
Such assertions are often made by the patients.
They keep their most important fancies and
reminiscences hidden for a time, and afterwards
insist emphatically that they have told us all
about them ; or they exclaim with an air of
innocence : " Didn't I tell you that before ? I
seem to remember distinctly having spoken to
you about it."

The patient next related to me the most
important factor in her condition—her belief
in the omnipotence of thought. Thought is
capable of inflicting the greatest misfortune !
This woman believed herself to be a particularly
gifted person. This belief in her greatness,
which now came to the surface, is what I have
named the neurotic's belief in "his great historic

mission." Without an appreciation of this trait in neurotics, no analysis can be complete. It is not enough for the patient to overcome his idea of his own "littleness," his feeling of inadequacy, his alleged inferiority; he must also learn to give up his belief in his unconquerable nature, the fiction of his "great historic mission." If he is cured through psychoanalysis, the cure probably indicates the first occasion on which the patient has allowed himself to be conquered, after which he is content to assume the modest rôle which he is destined to play in real life.

This patient afterwards decided when the treatment should end. She suddenly became desirous to return home. But she first intimated that there were still some things of which she wanted to free her soul. Finally she relented and told me the last phantasies she had been withholding during the entire period of the treatment. They showed that she had always held the belief that she would attract the attention of the higher powers through her exemplary abstemious conduct. The fancies of her youth had reacted upon her as an "eternal warning" to turn from the path of self-indulgence and to devote herself to a life of virtue. Her mind was chiefly concerned with the problem of eternal bliss. That was why she had been able for thirty years to endure a prisoner's life, locked in her room. For what does this short life amount to when contrasted with an endless eternity? Her sufferings were but a preparation for the highest bliss, and were to earn her a place in Heaven. In that other life she would triumph over all those who had devoted themselves to earthly pleasures in this. Her life was a preparation for the last triumph, and the feeling of dread would protect her against the chance of sinning.

Cures of this kind can be effected without psychoanalysis. I recall the famous case of the woman-sleeper of Oknö who maintained her dormant state for thirty years and then suddenly rose and went about her household duties. People flocked from far and wide to witness the miracle. This woman had undoubtedly been preparing herself for that historic occasion. Her whole life had been a preparation for that great miracle.* My patient, too, longed to be looked upon as a wonder. She told everybody that after thirty years of invalidism she had been cured by me, and that, after having been treated without result by sixty-three other physicians in succession.

* Fully explained in my Monograph, *The Will to Sleep*.

I wanted to introduce her to a medical association at one of its meetings, but on that particular day she had a fresh attack of dread and was unable to come to me unattended. That she begrudged me the triumph was shown by the fact that the very next day she went about the streets freely by herself. She juggled with her fears so skilfully that by their aid she dominated her whole family; she tried to press me into her service, too. Not succeeding in this, she gave up her anxiety, which did not return until the day when my triumph was to have become public. At the same time she confessed to me that it would have given her great satisfaction to have made her appearance and to have been admired as a " rare case." Suddenly, however, the thought had come into her mind : " You will not be an unusual case. You are an ordinary healthy person."

I have received from this patient a number of letters expressing her gratitude. She wrote me an account of her triumph. In Russia she looked up all the physicians who had treated her without result, and showed them that she was cured.

Then she wrote and asked me whether she had not better come to Vienna for a short visit in order to undergo an " after-cure." There were a number of important points she wanted to go over with me. I advised her not to do so. I pointed out that it was a lengthy journey from Riga to Vienna, and urged her to rid herself of the remains of her neurosis through her own efforts.

I was very astonished one day to see her enter my consulting-room. She then related the following occurrence : She had gone to a famous physician in Petrograd, and had told him about her wonderful cure. (This doctor had tried his own method of treatment on the patient without satisfactory results.) He gazed at her for some time and then said : " This Dr. Stekel must be a clever man." That remark had caused her to stop and think. " Do you know," she continued, " I once read about a patient who insisted that there was a bird in his head. A make-believe operation was performed on him, and he was shown a bird which he was told had been found in his head and removed. The patient got well. It has occurred to me that perhaps you have not cured me by the new method after all, but through suggestion, and that you have made me believe that I am well."

I looked at her for a moment in astonishment. The patient who had suffered from agoraphobia for thirty years, but was now well, had obviously returned to Vienna to get back her old trouble, and triumph over me.

" Can you go out by yourself freely ? "

" Yes."

" Have you any attacks of dread ? "

" No."

" Then what more do you want ? You can be glad that you are well. Is it not immaterial how you got well so long as you can walk about alone with no feelings of anxiety ? "

I explained frankly to her that she had returned to Vienna in order to punish me for my brief and business-like letters, by relapsing into her old agoraphobia.

The explanation worked wonders. In a few days she returned home perfectly satisfied and without a particle of her old anxiety left.

This case illustrates the sources of and pathway to success in psychoanalytic treatment. In psychoanalysis Freud has furnished us with a tremendous weapon : a weapon capable of inflicting terrific wounds if handled carelessly, but of inestimable value in fighting a neurosis if carefully used. Only we may have to modify many of our views, and we must guard against the tendency of appraising the value of the method merely on the basis of its current successes and failures.

IX

In the above case psychoanalysis helped me to uncover the root of the patient's feeling of guilt and acted as a mental release. But four months of treatment did not bring to light a single incident of which the patient had not been previously conscious. The reverse, of course, happens in some cases. But in this case it was only necessary to correct the patient's false-feeling attitude and the conflicts were clearly brought to light. The patient learned to speak and to think about phases of life about which she had previously been unwilling to talk or to think. She became aware of her death-wish for others, her criminal trends, her brutal egoism, her indolence, her envy and boundless selfish ambition. But she was cured only after she had given up her belief in herself as an " exceptional " being. The moment she had resolved to be an " ordinary " person the physician's task was accomplished. It is manifest that the chief task of psychoanalysis is to disclose the patient's resistance to treatment, and to convince him that he does not truly care to get well, that he is unwilling to give up the secret goal existing only in his phantasies.

I may illustrate this generalization by a quotation from the thoughts of Otto Ludwig. The creative writer knows what we physicians were for a long time ignorant of. The patient's belief in his " great historic mission " must be dissipated before he can find reality acceptable. Finally all psychoanalytic endeavours lead to the one aim—to reconcile the patient with the sober facts of reality. Ludwig expresses this thought very beautifully.

" Youthful idealism is vanity. With a certain measure of deliberation a young man turns his enthusiasm to any object which becomes linked with his vanity. And this feeling of vanity, to what more does it amount in the end than the lofty disdain with which the young man, in his deluded self-conceit, looks down upon everything real and human as something beneath him ? He requires the impossible of others, not because he is capable of accomplishing the impossible himself—not that—but because in his case he takes that for granted.

" Scepticism, which is a phase following the period of enthusiasm and grows out of the latter as its antithesis, is the great educational fever through which man's soul must pass, and the condition of its enlightenment. A man must learn to doubt his imaginary worth in order to

become certain of his real worth. What he
formerly expected of others without knowing
whether he himself could do it or not, this he
will now do without expecting it of others.

" His highest ideal was at first to die glori-
ously for something ; now his ideal is the
supreme one : to live humbly for something."

This is the final result which the psychoanalyst must from the beginning bear in mind.
He who has learned this secret holds the key to
the greatest possibilities of successful treatment.

X

There was a particularly sacred doctrine
advocated in psychoanalysis to the effect that
" the patient must take the lead." This rule
certainly has its justification. It would be
ridiculous to say : " To-day I will take up the
incest-complex, to-morrow I shall discuss the
problem of the relationship to the father," etc.
The patients should be ready for the definite
problems before they are taken up. The
experienced psychoanalyst can judge when the
proper time has come for discussing this or that
particular problem. But woe to the analyst
who permits the patient to take the bit between
his teeth without the least control, and who

looks upon the spontaneous associations of the patient as rulers in the field ! Thereby the gates are set wide open to wantonness, and it is in the patient's power to lead the physician by the nose, as it were, and to prolong the treatment *ad infinitum*. It is for the analyst to appraise the associations critically, and he must distinguish between what is useful and what merely arises on account of the resistance. He must know how to separate the grain from the chaff, and he must always be ready to step in at the proper moment. That is far from easy, because a sensitive patient is readily disturbed and always defends the significance of his associations with great stubbornness. Indeed, these defences are the channels through which he forgets his ingenious weapons of obstruction and passive resistance.

All the actual current events, upon which the patient is fond of dwelling, the letters from home and from his sweetheart, the exciting occurrences of the previous day, the endless dreams which are produced in unaccountable numbers, are so many manifestations of resistance : it is necessary firmly to limit these accounts to essentials, to ignore completely any theoretic objections to psychoanalysis, and, by an inflexible discipline, to put an end once for all to obstructions.

I may illustrate this in connection with a case of psychic impotence. A physician who ran away from women at the critical moment, or, at the most, accomplished *ejaculatio ante portas*, began a psychoanalytic interview by reading a letter he had just written to his bride, which was supposed to exhibit his bipolar attitude. I have heard dozens of such letters, and this time I refused to listen to it. The physician next recalled certain impressions which the reading of a case in the *Jahrbuch für Psychoanalyse* had made on him. I made short work of that, too. After a pause of a few minutes, the patient told me that, when he was a school-boy, he could not bear it when the teacher wrote on the blackboard with chalk. It gave him a physical sensation of discomfort, almost amounting to pain, in his teeth. His next association was that the sight of, and especially the stroking of, satin, had a similar effect, setting his teeth on edge, and it made him shudder when he passed his hand over a satin collar. His next association was that he was reminded of a friend who was hard of hearing.* One had to shout into the man's ears. But sometimes this friend would show a wonderful adroitness in " catching on." (I

---

* Referring to the analyst, who was so hard of hearing *that he failed to hear the things of most importance.*

mentally thanked him for the implied reproach and compliment.) The next thing he told me was that he had often regretted that he had not specialized as a gynecologist and particularly as a surgeon. In that connection there followed a long-drawn-out tale about a teacher who adopted the policy of searching his pupils' homes to discover whether they were hiding books of a forbidden character. (Again a reference to our inquisitorial rôle.) Next followed an animated account of the various High School teachers, which I recognized at once as mere " padding " and firmly put a stop to. I felt I should like to investigate the meaning of that particular idiosyncracy—his objection to the chalk-writing on the blackboard, and I asked the patient how he explained that in his own mind. He pondered a little and then said : " The chalk is a phallus symbol ; the board is the vagina." Now I assumed a tone of anger : " Do you consider me such a fool and simpleton that you dare to advance such an explanation ? "

The patient laughingly answered : " I confess frankly that I wanted to make fun of you. I thought that you, the symbolist, would certainly fall into the trap."

I then pointed out the connection between the idiosyncracy and the sensation in the teeth.

The chalk obviously symbolized bone, satin the " satin-like " skin, and that we probably had to do here with a case of the cannibalistic complex.

Suddenly the patient became loquacious. The day before he had discussed cannibalism for an hour. He had confessed to a number of sadistic phantasies, and had stated that they had played a great rôle in his childhood. He recalled something that had not crossed his mind for twenty years. He was a child of four or five when he heard the story of a butcher who was very famous for his "sweet hams," and carried on a very successful business. The story ran that this man had a trapdoor, through which purchasers, calling at odd times when no one else was by, disappeared into the cellar, where he himself murdered them. The human flesh thus acquired he used in the preparation of his goods, and that was what made the hams so " tasty " and sweet. (Such stories are told to children!) Another story of a man who devoured his sweetheart had also made a powerful impression on his mind. The old blood-accusation brought against the Jews came up for discussion and he confessed that he believed the Jews did use human blood. . . . In a word, important material flowed from his lips like water gushing from a newly opened spring.

On the following day he revelled in cannibalistic fancies. He was obviously bent on reducing my discovery *ad absurdum*, and represented himself in his phantasy as devouring his sweetheart piecemeal. He exaggerated his sadistic leaning towards women, and attempted to make it look ridiculous through exaggeration. There followed reflections of doubt concerning psychoanalysis. The associations might rouse forgotten complexes and thus lead to confusion. . . .

I explained to him that psychoanalysis does not create these complexes, that it merely brings them forward into the light of consciousness. He said he was secretly afraid of these instincts, and that was why he had never married. That was why he did not dare to go near a prostitute, he, for whom Jack the Ripper was a cryptic ideal. But through my treatment he hoped he might find that he had been afraid of mere shadows, that these phantasies would never crystallize into deeds. He hoped he might quietly examine the Medusa head and put the question at rest for ever. Every neurotic represents a regressive stage of existence in which the primitive instincts are immeasurably the strongest. But these instincts have long since been tamed and converted into moral standards. If he feels that he stands above these instinctive cravings he need have no fear, etc.

It is the task of psychoanalysis to unburden the patient's minds, to convince them of the harmlessness of their phantasies which often only scare them and hold them in check. They then use these childish phantasies in order that they may always possess a memento of their vileness, and they compare themselves with others, with the result that they become obsessed with a feeling of their own inferiority.

XI

I have already said that it is very difficult to induce a patient to abandon his fiction about his " great historic mission," and to modify his ideas of his own importance. The " *sentiment d'incomplétitude* " serves as a bipolar antithesis for protection against the urge of selfish ambition as well as a self-excuse : " You would attain the greatest position the world offers if you were not so weak and ill—if you were only in good health ! " The neurosis itself plays into the hands of this tendency to self-excuse and as a genuine reason for failure to accomplish anything great, i.e., as a counterpoise to self-reproach for achieving nothing and for the indolence which arises from the natural dislike of ordinary occupations.

The task of the analyst is to reconcile the patient to reality. With that end in view, the analyst must also be qualified to act as an educator; consequently the practice of psychoanalysis requires men of above the average capacity; they must be to a certain extent creative artists, capable of building up personalities. The analysis must be followed by synthesis, to use Dr. B. Martin's apt expression.

Naturally in such cases the patient looks upon his physician as the representative of authority, against which he has fought all his life, and in that struggle his illness supplies him with the most valuable weapon.

The old spitefulness now reasserts itself against the physician, and the treatment becomes either an open or a hidden struggle, in which the physician must be allowed finally to play the rôle of victor. I can only agree with Alfred Adler, who, as an experienced psychothera-peutist, declares : " As a last resort, after an exhaustive treatment, the self-sacrifice of the physician must be called upon ; he must assume all responsibility for his alleged failure to complete a cure. In two of my cases this subterfuge worked well ; one patient was healed by a Bosnian rural physician through correspondence, and another—a case of trigeminus neuralgia of several years' standing, in which in the course of two years, I had achieved only fluctuating results—was cured by waking suggestion. Often cases such as these, after the actual treatment has ceased, show marked improvement, enjoy long intervals of good health, and sometimes complete recovery."*

For these reasons it is very difficult to furnish statistics regarding one's therapeutic results. I have really very seldom heard patients say : " Doctor, I am well now—thanks to you ! " On these occasions the patient was generally far from cured, but said it merely as a subterfuge to put me off the track and to prevent my further searching of the unconscious. More often the patient is inclined to prolong the course of treatment, hoping thus to prove to the physician that his case is hopeless. Again, the treatment often has to come to an abrupt end. I once cherished the illusion of remaining the patients'

* Adler: *The Neurotic Constitution*, Authorized English Version by Dr. B. Glueck and Dr. J. E. Lind. London: Kegan Paul. New York: Moffat, Yard & Co. 1921.

friend, to guide them and advise them after the treatment, to see them from time to time and direct them on their proper path. To-day I know that it is best for those who are healed and for those who are on the way to being healed to bid a final farewell to the physician ; and I also know that sometimes it is best to bring about the parting abruptly, even at the cost of one's personal feelings. The abrupt ending of relations between doctor and patient is an excellent means of rousing the patient's feelings of spite.

I treated the serious case of a compulsive neurotic who had abandoned his studies for four years, although he was ready to take his doctor's degree. The treatment brought about no alleviation, although all his compulsive acts had been cleared up. The clearing was helpful only so long as the patient was obliging enough to yield to the analyst. I therefore wrote to his parents and warned them not to be surprised if I should drop their son's case ; that we might have a scene in the course of which I might show him the door. A few days later I thought that the time had arrived for me to stop the case. The patient was always " over-sensitive." I reproached him for not resuming his studies and for concealing his indolence. He gave a sharp and excited answer ; I retorted still more sharply, and that roused him to make a cutting remark. I used this as a pretext, and informed him that I had done with his case, adding : " The fact is, you do not want to get well, and now that I have withdrawn my assistance, you will not get well."

" On the contrary," was the excited retort. " I shall show you that I can get well without your treatment ! "

That is just what happened. He returned home, took up his studies again, received his doctor's degree, and—his equilibrium restored— afterwards made it up with me. Previous to that, I had met all his requests for forgiveness and for permission to resume the treatment with the most relentless and firm refusal.

The treatment of cases of impotence is more gratifying. The results are obvious. In such cases the patients themselves are anxious to be able to indulge in their *vita sexualis*. The " will to be ill " is more easily overcome and is displaced by the will to be well.

XII

Another important question is : Shall the ex-patient continue to be interested in the analysis and to preoccupy himself, for instance, with its literature ? Shall he be trained in psychoanalysis by us and be thereafter expected to free himself permanently of his compulsive and symptomatic acts and of his various newly developed symptoms ? Shall he become the physician of his own soul ?

This is a question towards which I have radically changed my attitude. I consider it a mistake to make psychoanalysts out of one's patients and to introduce them in psycho-analytical societies. I have never seen this course followed by such good results as when patients are encouraged to forget all about psychoanalysis and their troubles. It is not the function of psychoanalysis to convert neurotics into psychoanalysts. It is natural that most physicians should become psychoanalysts in that way, for many a one in trying to help others helps himself. Nietzsche says : " Psycho-analysis becomes for those physicians a calling and an aim. Unfortunately these psycho-analysts themselves remain anchored to their complexes—a condition I have designated as ' psychoanalytic scotoma,' the psychoanalyst's ' blind-spot.' " That may be the reason why so many bitter feelings are displayed between physicians, especially among neurologists and still more among psychoanalysts.* But we should endeavour to raise ourselves above our affects and to overcome our complexes. We must do so if we are to help others. But the neurotic will do well promptly to forget the analysis and everything pertaining to it, as soon as he is cured. Otherwise the psychoanalysis will only become a pretext for him to hold on to his neurosis. This may be seen particularly often in the case of compulsive neurosis. The apparently cured sufferers are no longer obsessed with their various compulsive images or acts, but they often become just as much obsessed with their dissolutions and explanations instead ; in short, their interest is still centred on their morbidly over-stressed complexes, with this only difference, that they now clothe their obsessions in psychoanalytic terms.

I have seen many such cases—neurotics who dreaded their incestuous wishes, where formerly they had been obsessed by a symbolized form of anxiety. So long as the patient is not free from

* It is never decorous to tell tales out of school. But even an inexperienced person after some intercourse with psychoanalysis must arrive at the conviction that most of Freud's younger pupils have scarcely applied the principles of psychoanalysis towards the removal of their own complexes. How much I had to endure as a member of the Vienna Psychoanalytic Society ! I hope some day to write the history of the psychoanalytic movement objectively and with care. I must wait until I can have the benefit of looking at the problem from a distance. According to reports which have reached me the situation does not differ from that in other places.

anxiety, we are not justified in speaking of a cure, even though he has become fully aware of the objects of his feeling of dread (incest, paraphilia, criminality). He must first raise himself above his complexes. That is also true of the feeling of doubt. I saw a man who had been treated for some time by Adler on account of a morbid feeling of doubt. He was in love with a girl, and doubted whether he was sufficiently potent, whether he could make her happy, whether he would be able to support her, and so on. He came to me with the statement that he was in love with a girl, but was all the time trying to "belittle" her ; he feared she would triumph over him and would always be above him. He could not bear to be belittled and " subject " ; that roused the " male protest " on his part and that was the reason why he was unhappy. He persisted in his feeling-attitude of doubt—but this time he had adopted the Adlerian mechanisms. Probably his feeling-attitude of doubt was due to his resistance to the physician, and that was the reason of his change of physician and why he had come to me. But this very feeling-attitude of resistance or contrariness, which had belonged originally to the father-imago, showed that his reactions were still morbid, and therefore in his case we could not speak of a cure.

The patient must cease to regard himself as a patient. He should put aside psychoanalysis and everything pertaining to it. He should not try to interpret dreams, or to ferret out symptomatic acts or solve obsessions. He should turn from himself and his psyche, and cultivate outside interests.

The longer he is preoccupied with psychoanalysis the more decisively will the latter assume in his mind the functions of his old neurosis. He reproaches himself when associations fail to come to his mind ; he fears that resistances are beginning to reassert themselves, and begins to doubt whether the physician is really helping him. This explains a remarkable fact. Certain cases grow worse the longer they are treated. The therapy of gonorrhœa has evolved a particular term with which to express overtreatment. Some cases of gonorrhœa fail to get cured because, through the treatment, the urethra is kept continuously irritated. Similar overtreatment may also take place in psychoanalysis. The longer a case is treated the more difficult becomes the final separation from the analyst. There are certain serious cases which do require a prolonged period of treatment of twelve months or even longer. But I confess frankly that after my earlier experiences I have adopted the policy of lessening the period of treatment very considerably, and allow a longer time for the most advanced cases only—for patients who are downright invalids and who have also experienced organic trouble. I do not usually suggest such a long period as a whole year, and endeavour to curtail it as much as possible. As I have already stated : those patients who have but a limited time at their disposal—physicians who have left their practice, employees who have been granted a limited leave, housewives whose presence is urgently needed at home—patients such as these give the best prognosis.

That may explain the fact that my results were so satisfactory at the beginning of my psychoanalytic practice. The period of treatment was short. I described some of the cases in my work, *Conditions of Nervous Anxiety*.

I now propose to go through the cases which I reported there, and to give a brief critical report of the final results of some of them. It is very difficult to obtain accurate data and to arrive at definite statistical facts. Many patients disappear entirely into the obscurity from which they had emerged. Of others one hears only incidentally and in round-about ways.

XIII

Looking over my results, I have reason to be very contented. I possess some information about most of the cases which I recorded in my *Conditions of Nervous Anxiety*. The singer (case No. 106 of the 2nd edition) is able to appear in public, to withstand the buffets of fate, and suffers only from minor neurotic disturbances from time to time. These are not serious enough to prevent her from striving and achieving in her chosen career. (Duration of treatment, four months, one half-hour to one hour daily.) Of the Rumanian priest (case 98) I had not heard for a long time. One day a lady came to me from Rumania suffering from agoraphobia. The priest (I. B.) had sent her to me. He had been very seriously ill, and a physician had cured him in Vienna with some simple drops. He had said this with a peculiar smile. She was merely to tell Dr. Stekel that he was perfectly well. She requested me to prescribe those miraculous drops for herself, and could not believe that I had cured the priest " only with talk." The treatment of this case lasted six weeks. And thus most cases get along fairly well, if fate does not press them too hard. Some have withstood even the most severe blows very successfully.

On the whole, therefore, I am justified in feeling fairly well satisfied with my results, especially when I add those cases which got well subsequently, ostensibly through another kind of "treatment," as, for instance, the singer, who after taking a tea-infusion prescribed by a quack, for two months, entirely overcame a troublesome nervous disorder which had interfered with his singing. I must again give as my emphatic opinion that a short period of treatment leads to the best results, particularly in the case of phobias. That, I surmise, is due to the fact that the shorter time renders the dissolution (that is the giving up) of the transference more easy for the patient and does not afford the opportunity for too great differences in the emotional tension.

We also come across some patients who, after having been under treatment for hardly a week, rush round and tell everyone they meet, that psychoanalysis has not helped them. A doctor who suffered from a severe compulsion-neurosis and was introduced to a medical meeting at Odessa as one of the failures (!) of psychoanalysis, had been under my care for only about a week.

I may mention a successful case : A young man suffering from various obsessions and severe compulsive mannerisms came to me once a week only, for about half-an-hour each time. It would be gratifying if I could achieve such excellent results in all similar cases. But a cure is not often brought about as easily as that. These patients are particularly proud of their illness and generate the severest resistances. (For the treatment, as I have repeatedly stated, resolves itself into a hard struggle between patient and physician.) Sometimes this is due to the fact that the analyst fails to realize he is being lead by the patient, and allows the latter to skim over the surface of things with his associations. Under such conditions, progress is hardly to be expected, and the treatment may go on for ever. If the compulsion-neurotic is allowed to take the lead, the treatment may last a year or longer—it might be for years or a lifetime. The patient intends to prove, thereby, the serious character of his illness. The doctor must have the courage to throw up the treatment, and to do so abruptly. This is the very class of patients likely to return every now and again for an hour or so's consultation, merely to get rid of this or that particular little symptom ; soon their old dread of losing something reasserts

itself, their morbid fear of verdigris, syphilis
(syphilidophobia), or some other obsession of
the most foolish kind—for instance, that the
book-shelf is poisoned. The patients mean to
prove thereby that the physician has not helped
them out of their difficulty at all, and that they
are as badly off as they were at the beginning.
I avoid these possibilities by sending off the
patients as soon as the treatment is ended, and
by reducing correspondence with them to a
minimum—in fact, I advise them to act as if
they barely knew me. A large number of them
obey the right impulse of their own accord, and
act thus without any special instruction. They
free themselves absolutely from the physician,
just as they should. Such patients forget their
physician readily, unless they present the evil
picture of the Judas-neurosis. In my work
The Language of Dreams (English version by
J. S. Van Teslaar) I have described the Christ-
neurosis on the basis of a number of illustrative
instances. By the side of this we also find the
Judas-type of neurosis. A patient of this type
once confessed to me during our very first
consultation that he had it in his mind to write
a drama about Judas. " He thought his
character was of a much more interesting type
than that of Christ. Judas had sacrificed

himself, and had by his act of treason raised Christ to a Godhead" the patient "could not but feel that Judas was the greater of the two." I at once recognized that that man was himself a Judas, and that he would act in accordance with his character towards me. He strongly resented the inference. His whole nature was, he said, steeped in gratitude and feelings of friendship. But at a critical moment in my life he played precisely the part of a Judas towards me.* Some of the patients of this type resolve to lecture on psychoanalysis after their treatment is over, so as to prove that it is good for nothing, a passing fad; and state that they intend to sue for the return of the money spent on the treatment. They write scurrilous articles and letters to newspapers, become the bitterest enemies of psychoanalysis, discover biologic foundations for the neuroses, and emphasize the hereditary factors—in short, they plan their revenge and deliberately seek, and actually hanker after, some opportunity to play the rôle of a Judas. Since a number of practising psychoanalysts are former patients of mine who have themselves submitted to psychoanalysis, the tendency to seek out schismatic differences and to become

* Cf. The chapter, "The Traitor," in my book *Unser Seelenleben im Kriege*. (Berlin : Otto Salle.)

antagonistic may be due partly to this Judas-complex, and the fault may not always be with the unfortunate neurotic. A skilful analyst should be able to uncover the potential Judas, and avoid a perpetration of deceptions by that type of patient. He predicts it so frequently, he proves it so often through the patient's symptomatic acts and dreams, that the latter, out of sheer contrariness, will fail to assume the rôle of a Judas, so as to prove his physician in the wrong.*

On the whole, it may be affirmed that psycho-analysis has proved itself superior to all other forms of psychotherapy, particularly in the compulsion-neuroses. Ordinary influences and explanations do no lasting good in cases of this type. And, if the psychoanalysis succeeds, the result is so convincingly plain, and it involves so radical a transformation of the patient's

---

* I recently had an amusing experience with a typical " Judas " —a physician. Of his own free will he read my *Nervöse Angstzus-tände* and told me every day that he had found himself reading something else. With that and with his coming just a few minutes late and leaving very punctually (not to give " himself away " freely) he indicated his spirit of independence. One day he told me that he had read through Jones' study of " Hamlet " at one sitting with great enjoyment ; a work no doubt greatly enhanced in value he thought, by its excellent translation into German. It turned out that he had confused Tausig, the translator, with a medical man, " Tausk " who had often attacked me and my methods of investigation. He admitted that he thought " Tausk " was really " Tausig." He also suddenly thought of going to Freud and later still the wish to be treated by Tausig played a great rôle in his " Judas " phantasy.

whole personality, that the psychotherapeutist is assured of the gratitude of the patient's whole family. At any rate the treatment of these severe cases is the touchstone of the psychotherapeutist's skill. The termination of the treatment, the freeing and overcoming of the patient's feelings, the adjusting of the latter to life and to reality, from which he had previously shrunk back, are tasks beset with difficulties and obstacles.

XIV

We must take up every case as if the whole riddle of the neuroses were to be unfolded before our eyes for the first time. This open-minded attitude has enabled me to arrive at new conclusions in the interpretation of dreams. I am not unmindful of the fact that we are but at the beginning of our knowledge in the investigation of dreams and of the neuroses. Much water will yet be poured into our old wine. But we shall be all the more sober for that, and, instead of the intoxication of victory, followed by the disillusions of the " morning after," we shall have the experience of tracing back the trail of truth with open eyes.

My statements should be taken in this sense.

They are also intended as a warning against the practice of psychoanalysis by persons who are not qualified by native gifts and capabilities.

I have the impression that there is already too much promiscuous practising of psychoanalysis. Analysis may be compared to a serious laparotomy. Psychoanalysis is a complicated science, and, to use a fitting expression of Riklin's, " the delicate structures of a neurosis should not be handled by rough and untrained fingers."

Every psychotherapeutist is inclined to prove his views by his patients' statements. But in the course of the treatment the patient learns his physician's jargon, and uses the terms he has learned from the latter when he attempts to describe his condition. That leads to serious errors about the methods and the findings in a given case.

I am reminded of the air-balloons with which children love to play. The neurotic, too, allows himself to be filled with our ideas and " air." He thus seems to be a substantial massive figure. But he bursts when overstretched or he gives off the surplus of air. Only the degree in which the new ideas, attitudes, and views are permanently retained is the test of the method and the proof of its success.

PART III

PSYCHOANALYSIS, ITS LIMITS, DANGERS AND EXCESSES*

The First Psychoanalytic Society
The Epidemic of Analysis
Superficial Conception of Analysis
Analysis of Crowd-instinct
Neurologic Training for the Analyst
The Analyst as Artist
Need of Intuition in the Practice of Psychoanalysis
How Psychoanalysis may be Learnt
Dangers of One-sidedness
Not every Neurotic is Curable
The Secondary, or Post-analytic, Repression
The Rebuilt Wall
How the Truth must be Accepted
Truth alone does not Cure
Analysis as a Social Game
Illustration of Post-analytic Repression
Psychoanalysis and Schizophrenia
The Possibility of Cure depends on the Willingness to be Cured
Concluding Remarks

* A Lecture given at the University of Chicago, May 25th, 1921.

PART III

PSYCHOANALYSIS, ITS LIMITS, DANGERS AND EXCESSES

THE suggestion for the founding of a psycho-analytic society came from me. It was I who suggested to Freud that our little circle should meet and discuss the new psychoanalytic problems. We had never expected an over-whelming success for the new science. We knew that we had a terrific struggle before us. For a long time we remained an " esoteric circle "—a little group. Thoughts were freely exchanged and no one can now trace precisely what he contributed and what he received.

I still recall the astounding impression created when at one of our Wednesday meetings I produced a book by a Swiss author, then unknown, who praised Freud's doctrines. An even greater impression was produced by the views of a leading Swiss psychiatrist who took the opportunity of referring to Freud's views in connection with a book he reviewed in the *Münchener Medizinische Wochenschrift*. We had thought ourselves isolated upon a psychoanalytic island and, as Freud's adherents, were accustomed to find ourselves held up to the scorn and ridicule of the scientific world.

Hardly two decades have passed since then, and I am now confronted with a psychoanalytic epidemic. For what is taking place in England and in the United States now is nothing less than that psychic epidemic which Hope, a bitter opponent to psychoanalysis, had predicted ten years before, when he described it as a psychic contagion induced by contact with the teachings of Freud. I should have every reason to be happy, but . . . If only there were no ' but ' and ' if ' about it. Psychoanalysis is capable of freeing the world from harmful moral hypocrisy, and of reforming our educational system ; it may even bring about a transformation of our whole social existence—provided it is properly understood and becomes part of ourselves, i.e., provided that it imbues our very being and that we act as persons who have been analysed to the depths of our soul.

Truths must penetrate into our very flesh and blood. They must penetrate our souls ; they must be accepted and inwardly digested so as to become part of ourselves. Unassimilated truths skim the surface and lend only a deceptive appearance of knowledge, which, in truth, is no knowledge, but merely a reflex, a shadow.

I have found that unfortunately this new science of psychoanalysis has penetrated the soul of the masses in an undigested state, that it remains detached, a foreign body, incapable of changing the old prejudices and attitudes, incapable of relieving the inhibitions and of bringing about a healthier way of looking at things.

Herein I see the greatest danger for the wonderful new science ; for that reason, and for that reason alone, I feel called upon to raise a warning voice. I fear the reaction that is bound to follow this epidemic—a reaction which will mean a terrible danger for analysis and for the progress of the science.

My conviction grows daily stronger that physicians and laymen alike understand but very little about the true nature of psychoanalysis, although they may have read a huge mass of analytic literature.

The two examples following are taken from my more recent experience.

An American physician, the head of a well-known sanatorium, came to me in Vienna in order to take a few days' course in psycho-analysis. No question about money. He would pay me any amount I might see fit to charge. But he had no time. I must give the instruction in telegraphic fashion. But when I required of him, not only a rather extended and exacting period of study, but also that he should be analysed himself and later treat a few cases under my control, he left disappointed and disgruntled at the tedious " red tape " of the Europeans.

The second example : After a lecture before the Neurological Society of Chicago, a very vivacious young girl called upon me. With notebook and pencil in hand, she sat down facing me and said laconically : " Please analyse me ! " She had believed in dead earnest that the analysis could be performed in the same summary manner as the extraction of a painful tooth. What she needed was an interesting article for the " Evening Post." Upon my explanation that such a procedure was impossible, she incredulously shook her dainty head and pouted : " You can if you will ! "

Various quacks, charlatans, and half-baked " professors " have already taken up psychoanalysis. In the United States there are analytic classes, conducted by layfolk and physicians, analytic sermons, nay, even analytic fortune-tellers. The Americans' interest in everything novel and curious is exploited to the discredit of psychoanalysis. A lady-physician in New York City gave six lectures on " How to become a millionaire through the aid of analysis." The recipe was very simple : You overcome your inhibitions ; energies formerly bound down are released ; and the path to success and fortune lies wide open before you !

Newspaper advertisements proclaim the virtues of books on self-analysis, compendiums are published, of 100 Questions and Answers, such as : " How to Acquire a Knowledge of Psychoanalysis in a Few Days " or " What Everyone should Know about Psychoanalysis " ; and books " All about Psychoanalysis " are recommended and eulogized.

There are already analytic hospitals and schools in England. Although I know that Freud warmly supports the idea of psycho-analytic classes for out-patients, I am decidedly against the plan. Analytic hospitals too, I consider senseless, ridiculous and even dangerous.

Whether the following little story is true I do not know, but it was told me by an English lady. At an English hospital for psycho-analysis a couple of patients discussed the serious nature of their respective troubles. The first woman patient called out triumphantly : " You, impertinent, healthy person—have you any idea of what I am suffering from ? Think of it ! I have the Œdipus-complex ! I am emotionally fixed on my father." " Oh, that is nothing," retorted the other ; " Look at me ! I am fixed on my father, two brothers, and my grandfather, and, besides that, I have other very serious complexes."

Analysis can never be suitable for group treatment. It must always remain an individual science. At the most, it may be possible to arrange for educational and corrective instruction in classes. Educational and sexual problems may be advantageously discussed in public to a certain extent, for the benefit of parents.

There are no classes for abdominal operations.

Analysis may be compared to a difficult operation, as Freud himself has pointed out. But an idea which has spread, particularly among the English-speaking public, confounds psychoanalysis with hypnotism, and places it on the same footing with waking suggestion. The analyst, according to this popular notion, amounts to a modern magician ; he is a person endowed with wonderful, supernatural powers, which enable him to uproot the disease in a couple of sittings. The analysis is compared to a mill into which the patient is put ill and suffering and from which he emerges healthy and strong.

Freud has compared analysis to an abdominal operation. But it is an operation that requires time and ever more time. Yet there are people who imagine that they have been subjected to psychoanalysis if they have spent a couple of hours with an analyst. I have repeatedly heard the remark : " I have been analysed. But it did me no good." Upon closer inquiry I have found that the so-called analysis had only lasted a few days. Analysis is a difficult educational ordeal, requiring time and patience. Truth alone does not accomplish the cure. I shall revert to this point later.

It is unfortunately a proven fact that not every physician is capable of becoming a psycho-analyst. Many general practitioners become interested in the new science, but only a few achieve mastery therein. The preparation for it consists of a thorough medical training and an accurate knowledge of neurology and psychia-try. I have met many psychoanalysts who had never been inside a psychiatric hospital in their lives. How should such a man be able to differentiate between the first stages of schizophrenia (dementia precox) and a hysteria, between somatic and psycho-sexual infantilism, between a compulsion-neurosis and a paranoia ? How should he be able to distinguish between organic and functional gastric disturbances, if he does not possess the basic knowledge for a true diagnosis ? Even the most experienced psychoanalyst makes mistakes sometimes. I myself once overlooked a multiple sclerosis in its early phases, and mistook the hysterical superstructure for the genuine trouble. Freud once mentioned to me that the same thing had happened to him. I recall a case of myasthenia which I failed to recognize during the first few days.

I call attention at this point to two cases published by me in 1911 in the *Zentralblatt für Psychoanalyse*, under the title " On Differential Diagnosis of Organic and Psychogenetic Disturbances." These cases were turned over to me by one of the most eminent analysts. *Homina sunt odiosa !*

Mr. N. B. was sent me by a physician of my acquaintance to be psychoanalytically treated as a case of hysterical amnesia. N.B., a travelling salesman, thirty-two years of age, had been found by servants lying unconscious on the floor of his room in a hotel at S. His wife was summoned by telegraph and arrived two days after the occurrence. Mr. N. B. had promptly recovered consciousness, but was totally devoid of his sense of orientation and talked incoherently. He did not recognize his wife. He did not realize until some ten days' later that his nurse was his wife. He then came to Vienna. I saw him about four weeks after the attack. Before the attack and for a brief period immediately thereafter there was found to have been total amnesia. It was diagnosed without difficulty as a neurosis. It was a clearly recognized case of anxiety-hysteria induced by the practice of *coitus interruptus* covering a rather protracted period and by psychic conflicts connected with his married life. The man had been suffering for a rather long time from nervous pains in the stomach for the alleviation of which even morphia was totally ineffectual. This is an important symptom in the case of psychogenetic (psychogenous ?) pains. The remedies in most common use for the alleviation of pain are as a general rule ineffectual, or produce an effect only in large doses, in which case they induce a state of intoxication. Hysterical headache, for example, is very rarely alleviated by Pyramidon, Antipyrine, etc.

I now learned that the patient had received some atropin from a stomach specialist. It was thought that remedy would certainly help him. He had taken the atropin during the entire journey and also on the day of the attack. Of this he still had a definite recollection. But at that point the amnesia set in.

The diagnosis was not difficult. It was a case of atropin poisoning, which is known to be productive of the protractive mental confusion and other severe psychic symptoms exhibited by this patient.

I declined to analyse the patient. In a week's time the condition disappeared without further treatment.

The second case is still more important. A woman thirty-four years of age, married twelve years, was sent to me to be psychoanalytically treated for " psychogenous depression." The lady was just coming from a sanatorium, to which she had been sent by a neurologist, Docent X., with the diagnosis: Melancholia. As I was too busy to treat her myself, I turned her over to a physician who was studying psychoanalysis under me at the time. He informed me that the case gave good promise of success ; that the conflicts were pretty clearly defined. She was indifferent to her husband, was rather cool toward him, while she idolized a brother of hers, and was enthusiastic about him only, his talents, his goodness and his beauty.   But my assistant soon informed me that the lady entertained thoughts of suicide which alarmed him. He was afraid to assume responsibility in so difficult a case.   I caused the lady to come to me and was willing to treat her personally.   The first days I spent in a thorough examination of her amnesia.   I discovered a fact that she had hitherto withheld from the knowledge of her husband, namely, that she had had no menstruation since her eighteenth year.   For the past two years however, there had appeared a slight glycosuria, which every dietary treatment was powerless to remove.   When the patient was excited sugar appeared in the urine, only to disappear except for slight traces when her calm was restored.   She confessed that a disagreeable growth of hair had appeared on her face during recent years, and that she had daily extracted the hairs with a delicate pair of tweezers. Although she had been very passionate during the first years of her marriage, she was no longer capable of sexual enjoyment.   She laid this at the door of her husband's insufficient potency. But she was forced to admit that her other attempts, such as onanistic acts, had afforded her no sexual satisfaction.   Something within her had become atrophied.

The psychic symptoms were a considerable amount of restlessness and excitability. There were also the well-known self-reproaches of persons afflicted with melancholy. She had made mistakes that made her superfluous in the world. She pitied her husband for having such a worthless wife. She had frequent attacks of insomnia, and wept at the slightest provocation. She was persecuted with thoughts of suicide, but she was unwilling to disgrace her husband and especially her brother by such an act.

The diagnosis was not difficult. Diabetes, hypertricosis, amenorrhœa, alteration of sexual enjoyment, impotence and psychic disturbances are in their totality indicative of hypophysis. Her husband stated that her face had become slightly altered. The lips and the tongue had perhaps become larger. The Rontgen photograph shows an enlargement and distention of the sella turcica. Diagnosis: hypophysic tumour. In view of the hopelessness of the condition and of the successful treatment of Vienna surgeons in the treatment of this malady, an operation was recommended to the patient.

Both cases indicate how important it is for psychotherapists to have an exact knowledge of organic illnesses and disorders. Furthermore, the similarity of the neurotic symptoms to certain forms of intoxication induced by alkaloids and inner glandular secretions force us to a recognition of the connection between organic and psychic. It will be the task of future biological investigation to complete the bridge between them.

How often I have had cases referred to mc for treatment with the diagnosis of hysteria, only to have to refuse them shortly afterwards because they proved to be cases of schizophrenia. How easy it is in such instances to accuse the analyst with causing the patient to become insane! This reproach is not uncommon; unfortunately it has a certain basis of truth, as we shall presently see.

It is precisely the psychoanalyst who is in a position to establish the differential diagnosis between neurosis and psychosis much earlier than the ordinary psychiatrist, since he probes more deeply into the patient's soul, and is compelled constantly to observe the most subtle reactions of the mind. But he must not be blind; he must not suffer from an " analytic scotoma," or blind spot; he must be thoroughly familiar with the clinical pictures; he must not only be a thinker, but an artist as well.

Analysis can never be a trade. It is a new science; its foundations are still in a state of flux ; its truths are not yet definitely established. As I have said before : it is not the method but the physician who heals. There are no analytic formulæ, no specifics applicable to all cases. Psychoanalysis more than any other science requires differentiation and sympathetic insight. It also requires another quality, which, unfortunately, is not possessed by every one—intuition. There is a great deal that cannot be put into words—that can only be divined. There is such a thing as an analytic instinct. But this analytic instinct is characteristic only of artistic, i.e. creative, minds.

Another requirement for the analyst is a comprehensive general culture, particularly an extensive knowledge of literature. Many psychic injuries originate from books. Many books have a determining influence upon mental development.

I generally ask patients the first day of the treatment what book has made the greatest impression upon them—who their favourite author is. The answer to this question is more instructive than a hundred others. One will answer : Raskolnikoff, a second will name a criminal novel, a third will say that no book has particularly impressed him, a fourth is still reading fairy tales, and a fifth only the newspaper.   The answer at once gives a picture of the patient's mental personality.

A most important qualification for the analyst is a completely unprejudiced attitude of mind.   He must not attach himself to one particular doctrine and neglect the teachings of other masters of psychoanalysis.

A certain Swiss leader of psychoanalysis gives a superior smile when my name is mentioned.   He claims that he does not need to read any psychoanalytic literature.   A famous Viennese psychotherapeutist said to one of my students : " I do not need to read anything that Stekel writes.   I know beforehand everything he has written or ever will write." . . .

I advise all my students to familiarize themselves with the different schools of thought, and to make use of anything they find of value anywhere.   There is no analyst and no psychotherapeutist from whom we cannot learn something useful.   Even the mistakes of others are full of valuable lessons for us.   I further advise my students to look upon each case as a *novum* and to be prepared for surprises.   Any new case may cancel our former conclusions.   Prejudice is the hangman of truth !

How may psychoanalysis be learned ?   It is difficult to acquire it from books.   The best method is to submit one's self to a competent analyst for a thorough analysis. But that is not enough. One should also analyse a few cases under the same competent guidance. I mean daily analysis; and the results should be gone over with the instructor, step by step. Unfortunately very few analysts have gone through such a training. Freud once wrote an essay on *Wild Psychoanalysis*, in which he pointed out the dangers of psychoanalysis when carried out by incompetent persons.

We have compared psychoanalysis to a major operation. A surgeon must have a thorough clinical training. What should we think of a physician who undertook a serious abdominal operation without proper surgical training? He could be sued for malpractice. Yet there are physicians and laymen who dare to take up psychoanalysis after reading up a few books by Freud and other psychoanalysts. Should psychoanalysis be blamed for what they are doing, for their failures? It is high time that our teaching institutions, our universities and medical schools should establish chairs for instruction in psychotherapy and sexual science, for the training of specialists.

The superficial character of analysis, as carried out in many countries, is incredible, because one

so seldom has an opportunity for checking up
the work of the analysts, and the latter are
clever enough not to publish their clinical
histories and analyses. What they do publish
are usually general statements and the remark :
" As my analyses have shown " takes the place
of the clinical record proper. But unfortunately I have often had occasion to see patients
who had been previously subjected to so-called
analysis, and I am always astonished to find how
inefficiently the work had been carried out.
Every analyst seems to ride some hobby. One
analyst is always ferreting out the Œdipus-
complex, and thinks he has discovered some
profound truth when he proves that the patient
has been in love with his own mother. Another
discovers the inferiority-complex everywhere,
whilst a third can find nothing but thwarted
ambition, or the male protest, and so forth,
not to mention the analysts who even at this
late hour pursue the trauma hunt, still believing
that the discovery of the trauma will cure the
neurosis.*

* One may speak of four analytic periods : First, the period of the
psychic trauma ; second, that of the Œdipus complex ; third, that
of anal erotism and libido distribution ; and fourth, that of the
castration complex. How is the castration complex to be recog-
nised ? There is great danger of overlooking it. Sadger, in his
excellent work, *Lehre von den Geschlechtsverirrungen*, gives the
following points for our guidance : The female pubic hair is a
substitute for the penis ! The biting of the nipple by the suckling

I have described the analysis as a contest between analyst and patient. I have pointed out elsewhere the significant manifestations of bipolarity, of the competing will-to-suffer and will-to-be-well; the rôle of the neurosis in the patient's mental life; its pleasure-value to the patient; the significance of ambition, in its double rôle as the will-to-power and the will- (or instinct-) to-self-debasement; the patient's over sensitiveness, his psychic anaphylaxis, the rôle of religious emotions, etc.

The carrying out of a true analysis is an artistic piece of work; it can be accomplished only by skilful hands.

Even the Freudian school has at last been compelled to recognize "active psychoanalysis." The theory that we must analyse, without influencing the patient, leaving the latter to pursue his own course—an attitude which Freud has stubbornly defended for many years— is unworthy of a science which aims at calling

---

babe represents the later castration. The same ominous meaning is ascribed to the pulling off of the arm or leg of a doll. Further, I quote literally : " Symbolic castration is meant by the playful breaking of twigs, matches and tooth-picks, the breaking of cigar-tips and the plucking of flowers. Likewise the manicuring and clipping of the nails, cutting notches into trees and benches, and any sort of vandalism." Further, quoting literally, " It is a girl's lifelong reproach to her mother that she brought her daughter castrated into the world." ` Needless to say that such utterances not only are facetious but make psychoanalysis ridiculous and do it much more harm than good.

itself psychotherapy. The physician must be the patient's educator, and point out to him the path to useful activity and health ; with kind but firm hand he must turn him away from the realm of his useless phantasies and train him to carry on his work ; he must hold up before him the mirror of his dreamy inactivity, thus revealing his inner will to suffer, and spurring on his energies.

Not every physician is competent to become a psychoanalyst ; nor is every neurotic suitable for analysis. Please note : I reserve analysis for severe cases, for subjects who have become unable to live reasonable lives or to continue their work. For this reason, I am strongly opposed to the suggestion that every one should be analysed. I have often come across this opinion here and in the United States. The idea seems widespread that it is desirable for all persons to " take some analytic treatment " that they may be better able to withstand the struggle for existence and to feel more happy. I consider the analysis of a healthy person mischievous. Many persons are much happier with their wilful blindness and their neurotic attitude than when they are robbed of their illusions. The analyst has no right to be a fanatical apostle of truth at all costs. *Truth is*

not always a sure foundation for happiness.
Fictions are often a much firmer and better
foundation than the truth.

There are people who go to pieces when their
eyes are opened, and they are thus robbed of
their neurotic fictions. They are like a man
who has had cataracts removed from his eyes
and cannot endure daylight except as he gradually
becomes used to it. Moreover, we must not
forget that the neurosis itself is a healing
process, and that the neurotic repressions represent so many scars that cover deep soul-wounds
and that only dire necessity should place the
surgical scalpel in the psychoanalyst's hands.

I am, therefore, not in favour of laymen reading
scientific psychoanalytic literature. This is an
important consideration at a time when every
high school girl and college boy is carrying under
his arm a volume of Freud and a promiscuous
variety of other analytical books. Of course, I
refer here to the technical portion of the
literature, and not to the popular books, of which
I have myself written a number and which are
expressly intended for general reading. The
latter are all that is needed for the general lay
reader ; they orientate without doing any
harm ; they even do some good at times ; but
the purely medical works cause only confusion

in the lay mind, and furnish the sort of half-knowledge which may prove very dangerous indeed.

There is, in fact, a repression which may be much more dangerous than the neurotic repression. I call it "*the secondary, or post-analytic, repression.*" I refer to the kind of post-analytic repression,—experienced by a neurotic after his hysterical unwillingness to see has been removed, and his repressions have been made conscious with the help of the analysis. He assumes the rôle of a healthy person, who has overcome his complexes, and yet retains his old attitude, with the only difference that he has now more successfully concealed the latter from his consciousness.

I shall refer again to the great dangers of this post-analytic repression. I may illustrate the whole process by an example which will make the matter clear. I once heard a story which seems to me to illustrate the nature of this secondary repression very well.

Two sisters lived in a quiet, isolated home, protected and safeguarded by their parents. They were not wealthy ; they worked with a will. They were happy in their humble home. The only thing that disturbed them was the presence of a huge wall that rose in front of their windows, shutting out the sunlight and cutting off their view of garden and street. A bit of blue sky was all that shone into their humble home. Parents and children had often discussed among themselves the advisability of buying the neighbouring property and demolishing the wall. The parents died. The sisters saved, little by little, in order to secure a brighter outlook into the beautiful world outside. They were forty years old by the time they had saved enough to buy the ugly wall, and to have it removed. But the expected happiness did not materialize. The view from the window brought them no joy. There was too much light; too many ugly objects in the street met their eyes; they longed to have their beloved old wall back again. So they saved up their money for another ten years, had the old wall restored to its place, and were once more contented and happy.

Likewise many a neurotic sacrifices labour, time and money in order to be cured of his neurosis, i.e. to demolish the heavy wall which obstructs his view of the world and limits his mental horizon. For all neurotics suffer from a concentric shrinking of their mental field-of-vision. But all neurotics are not capable of enduring the larger vision which comes to them. After the analysis many, very many, of them painfully gather together the same old stones and build their second wall.

It is not enough for a neurotic to perceive and understand the causes of his illness. He must also have the will-to-be-well. He must receive the truth as part of his very being, not merely as an intellectual concept. The truth must pervade his inner self; it must become part and parcel of his fundamental personality.

The patient must be trained to that end. He must be lost to his neurosis and won back to life. He must become so immune through the wisdom acquired by the analysis that a secondary infection will be impossible.

That, unfortunately, is known to very few physicians. A mere intellectual recognition of the causes of the neurosis is of no avail against the neurosis itself. The neurosis is a disturbance of the emotions. A new emotion must be mobilized against the neurotic affect, against the "overstressed idea." In many cases, emotional transference to the consulting analyst renders that service. For that reason the building up and the releasing of the patient's transference is the analyst's most difficult and most important task.

I am reminded of the mistakes I made in the first years of enthusiasm over psychoanalytic discoveries. A man came to me complaining of all sorts of distressing symptoms, especially of the irritability towards his sister, with whom he was always quarrelling. He was subject to insomnia and sexual impotence while the victim of violent nocturnal erections. His sister, who had come with him, complained that he was always seeking a new quarrel with her, but that whenever she wanted to leave the house he was unhappy and broke into tears. She said he was jealous and kept her from meeting with other men. She also admitted that she tormented her brother with her own jealous fears, although these were groundless.

I gave them both to understand that it was a case of incestous attachment on both sides, and advised them to live apart. They both recognized that I was right. There were too many proofs to permit of denial. The man had often dreamed of intercourse with his sister, and she, in turn, admitted she had had similar thoughts and dreams. I made the bad mistake of eliciting this admission without analyzing the man sufficiently to ascertain the other causes of his neurosis. I had hoped that the separation of brother and sister would be followed by a complete victory over the incestous attachment. A few days later I received a letter saying they had talked over the matter thoroughly and come

to the conclusion that I was on the wrong trail,
that their thoughts of incest were due only to the
false teachings of Freud, whose books they had
been reading, and they now realized that the
whole thing was only the result of suggestions
conveyed by the reading of misleading literature.
The brother went away to a sanatorium and the
sister to the home of a female relative. After
four weeks they came together again. Some
months later the man attempted suicide after an
effort to outrage his sister—an effort alleged to
have been made in a state of dream. As I was
informed by the sister, whom I later treated with
success, he had played with her in all sorts of
ways when they were children, and had attempted
intercourse with her when he was seventeen.
The brother was successfully analysed by another
physician. Both have since married and are
mentally well poised.

For the acceptance and endurance of any
analytic truth the patient must be adequately
prepared.* For that reason I never offer any
explanations or solutions during the first hours
of analysis, even to persons introducing themselves to me as experienced analysts. Of course,
such persons assure me that I may tell them

* In most cases the patient accepts the truth in deference to the
physician, and regardless of his own feelings.

anything, that they have studied the whole subject of analysis, etc. But caution is to be advised—even when dealing with physicians trained in analysis.

I treated a boy brought to me by a very intelligent physician who had read books by Freud and Stekel, and asserted he had successfully completed many analytical cases. He expressed the opinion that the boy was in love with his own sister. The analysis brought out the fact that he had actually been having intercourse with her for years. After a time the father came to Vienna to talk with me about the progress of the case. I declined to reveal any of the facts confided in me in the analysis. He called in the boy :

" You will allow the doctor to tell me everything, won't you ? Of course, you know my liberal attitude of mind."

The boy said : " I don't want to have any secrets from my father. Tell father the unvarnished truth."

Then I very reluctantly informed the father, in his son's presence, of the sexual intercourse of his two children. (The daughter was a year older than the son.) The father was very astonished, but remarkably composed and gave me a very interesting discourse. According to his liberal ways of thinking, incest was nothing unnatural, and he saw no harm in it, especially as the children had kept it up for the past five years, that is to say, since childhood. He then asked my advice as to the proper measures to take in the matter. I advised the permanent separation of the children.

I must confess I was astonished at the composure and broadmindedness of the father. The next day the boy came to me in tears. His father had beaten him unmercifully, threatened to disinherit him, called him a criminal and a dirty pig, and decided to have the analysis discontinued, as the boy was unworthy of analytic treatment.

As I learned later, it was jealousy that had so aroused the unprejudiced father. He had an incestuous attachment to his daughter himself, and regarded his son as a rival. Hence his brutal beating of the boy. His whole intellectual attitude had broken down and he behaved like every father who has no knowledge or experience of infantile sexuality.

Every analyst knows that neurotics who have read everything bearing upon psychoanalysis that they have been able to lay their hands on, are particularly difficult to cure. But it is not so well known that the knowledge of conflicts and emotions thus gained is used by these neurotics as a means of playing hide-and-seek with themselves : and of becoming still more deeply enmeshed in the network of the neurosis.

All attempts at self-analysis usually suffer failure because of the tendency of the unconscious to protect itself by means of secondary repression against further probing. Public analyses are even more dangerous. The analysis is too important and too penetrating a procedure to be used as a social game, in which one person interprets another's symptomatic acts. Dream-analysis, too, is far from being a harmless pastime. The analysis of dreams is a scientific medical procedure ; only in exceptional cases may it be permitted to give tentative interpretations.

There is always the danger of secondary repression, the latter often raising problems that the analyst finds most difficult, and, unfortunately, at times unsolvable.

Whilst in the United States, last year, I was asked to treat a young woman who was suffering from all sorts of neurotic symptoms, including depressions and inability to concentrate on any mental task. She was a member of a circle which had devoted much attention to psychoanalysis ; in it books by Freud and others had been read and discussed. Her behaviour in my presence seemed very peculiar. She said :

" I am really well. I believe that if I had sexual intercourse I should be rid of all my symptoms."

The impression she made, in other ways as well, pointed to a rather serious mental dissociation; so that I hesitated in my diagnosis between schizophrenia and hysteria. Some of her statements struck me as so strange, that I came to the conclusion that she was posing and that she was not truthful. At the very next appointment I began the interview with the question :

" Why did you play the actor yesterday while talking to me ? "

" I do not know why. But it is true that I did. . . Something I cannot explain impelled me to try to mislead you.

But presently another personality unfolded itself. She became her usual, ordinary self again, and then confessed that she had secretly married. Neither her parents nor the husband's had any knowledge of it. But, although they were man and wife, they had not come together. They had no home of their own, or any other place where they could be by themselves.

Some discrepancies in her statements, even

then, led me to doubt her alleged great affection for the young man. She could not tell me enough about "Jacques,"—her husband—about his wonderful qualities, or of her consuming love for him. The fact that he was not yet earning twenty-five dollars a week was the only thing that stood in their way and prevented their setting up a home. He only earned twenty dollars a week and she herself had a very good position. This explanation seemed to me as untrustworthy, as the reasons she had already given as to why they could not be together—a thin and transparent mask to conceal her inner aversion against the intimacy of married life.

I found out that her father knew about this love affair ; he was not opposed to it but had made the condition that she should submit to analysis by me before he would give his consent.

Recognizing an obvious "neurotic dodge" I said to her : You have assumed the defensive. You have run off and married the man, lest your analysis should discover that you do not love the young man after all."

She admitted it. I did not fail to note that she had anticipated a number of psycho-analytic questions and had prepared herself in advance to meet them in her own way. Among others, the question came "Was she emotionally attached to her brother and in love with him ? " A dream which she had had a few nights before secretly marrying her husband pointed clearly in that direction. She had dreamed of intercourse with her brother, with whom she was deeply in love. That brother had married a few months before and had made his home with his parents. But she used her psychoanalytic knowledge to bring about a secondary repression. She had said to herself : " My brother is merely a substitution, a surrogate. He stands for his friend, Jacques. I dreamed of intimacy with Jacques."

That case was lost to psychoanalysis. For the girl's love for Jacques was only imaginary. But the marriage was a fact which had to be taken into earnest consideration. Therefore, I gave up the analysis and advised her to inform her parents of what she had done. The parents arranged a home for the couple and made the marriage public. I told the girl's mother that I could not hold out a favourable prognosis for the future ; that I had to regard the marriage as a symptomatic act, the consequence of a secondary repression.

Unfortunately my prognosis proved true, only too soon.

If this young woman had come to me without any knowledge of psychoanalysis, the analysis would have been the means of her finding out for herself that her infatuation for Jacques was a displacement, a substitution, Jacques, her brother's friend, serving merely as a surrogate for her hidden emotional attachment to her own brother.

The secondary repression is much more troublesome than the primary. In psychoses I have often observed some truth pressing into consciousness just before the outbreak of the psychosis. Perhaps these facts bring us a little closer to the understanding of the psychoses. I have not the least doubt that an unsuccessful repression may lead to a more complete dissociation. For that reason an unsuccessful analysis may be a source of danger to the patient. He knows too much for comfort and not enough to be well. He is impelled to carry out a renewed, stronger repression ; he ignores more completely than ever a certain portion of reality ; and takes deeper refuge in the world of phantasy. He builds a second wall around his spiritual self. The psychosis is the victory of infantilism over reality.

Many psychiatrists claim that they have seen schizophrenia develop after analytic treatment.

I have been informed by a Swiss analyst that he saw ten such cases in one year.   On the other hand, that particular doctor carries out a sort of partial psychoanalysis.   Nevertheless I do not hold that the analysis produces the schizophrenia.   Such an assumption would be ridiculous, especially since schizophrenia undoubtedly has its own endogenous causes.   But an unsuccessful analysis may at times hasten the outbreak of the mental disorder, whilst a successful analysis may postpone the outbreak.   Undoubtedly psychoanalysis is capable of accomplishing wonders in certain emotional psychoses ; but unskilful management of the analysis may also be responsible for aggravations and set-backs.

Finally, we must have the courage to acknowledge that we cannot cure every case that presents itself.   The analytic art, too, has its limitations ;   it cannot, for instance, always deal successfully with the stubborn instinct of self-abasement manifesting itself in the will-to-suffer.   Cases of psychosexual infantilism prove particularly stubborn.

We simply have to face the unpleasant fact that we cannot cure every case, even when we employ the most correct and effective methods. There will always be incurable patients who, in their search for health, run from one analyst to another. These are among the patients who submit to analysis here, there and everywhere in order to justify their illusory belief that they are doing everything in their power to get well, when, as a matter of fact, they are all the time under the dominion of the will-to-suffer. It is no easy task to lure a man lost in day-dreams from the luxuriant realm of his phantasy into the dreary waste of a work-a-day world of reality.

We must take into account also the neurotic's hidden pride in his belief that his is a difficult case—one of the most baffling cases ; that he is alone in his misery ; that no other person is in quite such a plight ; and, above all, we must not forget the patient's hidden gratification at the thought that nobody in the world, not even the most famous specialist, is able to conquer his trouble. It is particularly difficult to prevail upon persons suffering from psychosexual infantilism to give up their fixed ideas and pet notions.

Often death is the best physician, freeing the sufferers from a psychosexual serfdom from which they are unable to free themselves either through their own efforts or with the aid of a physician. For that reason, we often observe unexpected cures following the death of a parent or of some other close relative. The case of paranoiac insanity reported by Bjerre as cured through analysis may owe the cure to something more than the mere treatment. During the analysis the patient's father died. That may have contributed considerably to the cure.

The fact is, there are some patients in a state of readiness to be cured, and others in a state of readiness to remain ill. The first case of paranoia, which I have reported in full in my *Psychosexual Infantilism* (authorized English version by Dr. J.S.Van Teslaar), was undoubtedly in a state of readiness for successful treatment. The very fact that the patient became engaged to be married shows that he willed to free himself from his infantile fixations.

Every reader of my larger works probably gets the impression that I appraise very highly the value of psychotherapy and particularly the practical worth of psychoanalysis. I do not hesitate to apply it even to psychoses, particularly paranoia. Nevertheless, I do not indulge in the illusion that I have found a panacea. I am fully aware that there are cases, in themselves curable, which the most thorough analysis on my part would not relieve.

Therefore it behoves us not to hold out a positive promise of cure. We can speak only of the possibility of a cure, and we must always point out that the case depends on two factors : the physician and the patient.

I must lay stress upon these facts because the over-estimation of psychoanalysis is fraught with great danger to the science itself, and because a superficial conception of its problems leads to the kind of analysis that is conducive to a secondary repression.

There is altogether much too much irresponsible talk about psychoanalysis carried on in public and in the press. There is already manifest, here and there, a condition we may call " analytic neurosis." This " analytic neurosis " is the result of overfeeding on second-rate psychoanalytia pabulum. We must not forget that blindness is a need. What should we say of anyone who could never drink a glass of water without thinking of the microbes and the infusoria that he had seen under the microscope ? Such a person would soon find life impossible. Life requires a certain amount of deception : it involves a certain degree of blindness. The philosopher's " thing in itself " is for most persons the thing which they do not want to see, and which they must not see. The analyst finds himself compelled, by reason of his professional duties, eventually to uncover the " thing in itself," and to expose it fully before the patient. But he does so only to enable the patient to recognize the truth, gain his health, and lapse again into a new world of quasi-deception.

I trust the reader will not misunderstand me. The more I revere and admire the splendid art of psychoanalysis the more I tremble for its future. I wish every physician who practises analysis to be fully aware of his great responsibility. We are all human and subject to error. Anyone may make mistakes and stray from the right path. But we must resolve to overcome our mistakes and to learn through our failures and errors.

We need schools for psychoanalysis and students earnestly bent on learning. We teachers must keep our pupils out of the paths of error. We must also protect the sufferers from exposure to unskilful and inexperienced advisers.

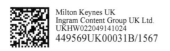

Milton Keynes UK
Ingram Content Group UK Ltd.
UKHW022049141024
449569UK00031B/1567